MW01519549

Eating for Good Health and Pleasure

Using the Food Pyramid and Food Guide to Your Advantage

Agnes M. Huber, Ph.D., R.D.

VANTAGE PRESS
New York

FIRST EDITION

All rights reserved, including the right of
reproduction in whole or in part in any form.

Copyright © 1996 by Agnes M. Huber, Ph.D., R.D.

Published by Vantage Press, Inc.
516 West 34th Street, New York, New York 10001

Manufactured in the United States of America
ISBN: 0-533-11551-5

Library of Congress Catalog Card No.: 95-90355

0 9 8 7 6 5 4 3 2 1

To my family for their encouragement
in writing this book

To my former students in their
counseling efforts

To the public who wants to get
the best from their daily food

Contents

Foreword

What an enormous pleasure it is to know that readers of this fine book have one of the finest minds in nutritional sciences at their disposal to simplify, rather than complicate, the process of choosing healthful and tasty foods every day.

Dr. Huber, who is an Oxford and Harvard graduate and a consummate nutritional scientist, is also one of the most approachable and humanistic people I know. Therefore I was not surprised that her book was so lucid, sound, and fun to read.

Let me tell you a little about the breadth of knowledge of this remarkable author. I first knew Dr. Huber when I was a student over two decades ago at the Harvard School of Public Helath, where she was on the faculty. Her lectures on the physiology and biochemistry of absorption were models of lucidity, just as the present text is. Dr. Huber's subsequent work, as senior nutritionist at one of the oldest university affiliated centers for children with special developmental and health needs, the Eunice Kennedy Shriver Center, and her later long and fruitful tenure as professor at Simmons College's department of nutrition further honed her counseling and education expertise. Thus the reader gets everything, from a deep understanding of the fundamental knowledge and biology, through to eminently sensible and practical tips.

I like this book because it is the kind one can give to friends and family and be sure that it is not only absolutely accurate, but also sensible and sensitive to individual differences. Dr. Huber proves again that taste and health can be partners, and that they do not have to be adversaries.

This will simplify my gift giving, and readers' eating!
Bon appétit.

—Johanna Dwyer, Sc.D., R.D.
Director Frances Stern Nutrition Clinic, New England Medical Center. Professor of Nutrition, Tufts University Schools of Medicine and Nutrition; 1994/95 President Elect, American Institute of Nutrition.

List of Figures

List of Tables

Acknowledgments

I wish to express my thanks to
Fiora Houghteling, M.Sc.,
Franz Huber, M.Sc., and
Elfriede Walz, nutrition instructor,
for their many helpful comments
and their encouragement

Eating for Good Health and Pleasure

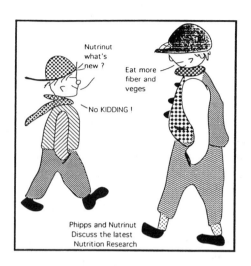

Chapter I
Gearing Up for the
Twenty-first Century

If you eat three meals a day and live to the ripe age of eighty, you will have eaten more than 87,000 meals. If you allow twenty minutes and spend $1.50 for each meal, you would take more than six years of your waking hours at mealtime at a cost of more than $130,000. Conservative estimates like these show the staggering amount of time and money we spend on our daily food, and we need to ask ourselves: Do we really get our money's worth?

But even if you are among the affluent with money and leisure and you are lucky to have plenty, there is still your health to consider. Nutritious food is a prerequisite for good health. It can make the difference between suffering chronic disease or leading a healthy life. The choice is up to each of us, and we need to learn to make informed decisions.

Diets that allow us to develop our full potential are not difficult to prepare. They use everyday foods from supermarket shelves and often are cheaper, especially if basic ingredients are used for their preparation. Often the difference between healthful diets and questionable practices is small and may not seem significant. Just consider the example of one 100-Cal cookie eaten daily *over and above* your energy need. The extra calories from this seemingly insignificant extra food will increase your body weight by ten pounds in one year and eventually lead to obesity. Healthful diets provide us with the nutrients and calories we need, give us a sense of satisfaction, well-being, stamina, and also lifelong health benefits.

Your Health: Product of Genes and Environment

Although healthful diets are critical, other factors are important also. The marvellous versatility in human nature, for example, is to a large part determined by the genes we have inherited from our parents. The color of our hair, the proportion and expression of our face, and the myriad other details that make us

2

unique depend on our genes, the blueprints locked in each of our body cells. That we become humans and not plants or animals depends on these genes.

The need for essential nutrients that must be provided by our diets is also determined by genes. All humans require the same types of vitamins and the same mineral elements, and every human being has a need for energy, which must be provided by a dietary mixture of carbohydrates, fats, and proteins. Slight individual differences in our genetic makeup affect our nutrient requirements to some degree, but all humans, except for those with certain rare genetic diseases, have the same obligatory requirement for energy and essential nutrients.

While the basic nutrient requirements are genetically determined, our lifestyle, including our dietary practices, also affects us. Whether we get enough sleep and exercise, whether our life is satisfying or stressful, whether we consume healthful diets throughout life, or whether we live on junk food will have consequences and affect how we feel, how healthy we are, and how we face life's challenges. It is scary and at the same time wonderful to have so much influence in shaping our own destiny and to influence who we are going to be.

That we have a choice is an awesome responsibility, for it is not immediately obvious what the best lifestyle should be for each of us. We are different by nature and cannot simply follow faithfully the suggestion of somebody else. We need to find out what is best for us specifically, how much sleep we require and the type of diet that is best to sustain our daily activities and keep us healthy. We need to find the appropriate exercise level our body needs and how much stress we can bear without getting depressed.

Modern Man in the Body of Caveman

The quest for a healthy lifestyle can be problematic since our own physical makeup has not adapted to modern life. It may sound incredible that the fashion model on the cover of a magazine, the Wall Street banker in his pinstripe suit, and the athletic-

3

looking football hero underneath their finery have the body of a caveman/woman. While our environment has changed drastically, our hearts, livers, guts, and brains, are remarkably similar to those of our ancestors thousands of years ago.

What has changed during the course of history and the development of modern civilization is how we conduct our lives. Two problems in particular have accompanied these changes, which have had serious consequences on our nutritional well-being and health. The first is progressive inactivity. No more hunting and foraging for food. Very little hard and long daily physical work. Eventually this drastic reduction in the activity of people in all walks of life has culminated in what some have called "the chronic couch potato syndrome."

The second change that has had far-reaching effects on our health, particularly in highly developed countries, is the overabundance of food and the dietary changes accompanying it. While our ancestors were used to active lives and frugal diets, we have become inactive and enjoy an overabundance of food. Such counterproductive changes have affected our health and our bodies have rebelled. Inactivity and dietary changes have had a serious impact on the well-being of modern man. They have resulted in premature chronic disease, such as heart disease, stroke, diabetes, obesity, and some cancers. There is no doubt that such disorders are of multifactorial origin, since genes and environment both are involved. However, diet specifically as well as physical inactivity are environmental components that are significant factors in their development and also in their prevention.

Changes in dietary patterns among fifteen countries, including the United States, involved in an international collaboration indicate global nutrition trends unfavorable with respect to such chronic diseases as cardiovascular disease, stroke, hypertension, and cancer.
   —B. Millan, et al., *Nutrition Reviews* 52 (1994): 201–7.

You Are What You Eat

The recognition that lifestyle and diet are causally related to the development of diseases plaguing affluent populations was first made in the sixties by two doctors working in Africa. They made the interesting observation that several diseases rampant in the United States and other highly civilized countries were virtually absent in the indigenous African population. Comparing the diets of Africans with those consumed in the United States, several significant differences were observed. For one, the content of fiber was significantly higher in diets of Africans. Their startling observations eventually led Drs. Burkitt and Trowell to hypothesize that diet and lifestyle are critical in the cause of these disorders. They suggested that heart disease, diabetes, stroke, obesity, and certain cancers are *Diseases of Civilization.* Recognition that environmental factors contributed significantly led to entirely new approaches. The new goal now emphasized their prevention. If these diseases are in large part a consequence of our dietary habits, their prevention should be possible by appropriate dietary and lifestyle changes.

"Nutrition is involved to some extent in almost all of the processes of human life. It clearly plays a role in the majority of the chronic degenerative diseases that cripple and kill most people in the United States."
—Special Report, Food and Nutrition Board, Institute of Medicine, National Academy of Sciences: *Journal of Nutrition* 124 (1994): 763 © J. Nutr. (124, 763), American Institute of Nutrition.

The Scientist's Story

For almost a century, nutritionists have studied how diet affects our health. Ever since the beginning of this century, studies were carried out to define the specific nutrient needs of children and adults. This extensive and often difficult research has led to the formulation of the Recommended Dietary Allowances (RDA), the nutrient requirements for people of all ages, which are the best data we presently have to allow us to make considered recommendations for nutrient adequacy. The RDAs are periodically updated as new scientific discoveries are made. They are used in national and regional nutrition surveys, and also for the assessment of the nutrient status of individuals. A diet providing nutrients similar to the RDAs is one with low risk for nutrient deficiencies.

Furthermore, based on the RDAs, in the early seventies, the U.S. RDAs were developed. The U.S. RDAs are the highest RDAs of each age and gender group. They have been used by food manufacturers in the past on food labels to educate the public on the nutrient and calorie content of foods. Nutrition labels on foods were introduced in accord with guidelines specified by the Food and Drug Administration (FDA). These labels were one of the first attempts to make nutrition information available nationwide.

Knowledge about essential nutrients, their function in the human body, and their food sources gleaned from scientific research during the first part of this century had a significant impact on dietary practices and consequently affected the health of adults and children in the United States. The devastating nutrient deficiencies such as pellagra (due to niacin deficiency) or goiter (from iodine deficiency) became diseases of the past. The discovery of their eradication by improving diets makes fascinating reading. It is but all forgotten that during the early twenties many inmates of New York's mental institutions succumbed to pellagra, the four Ds (dermatitis, diarrhea, dementia, and death). The discovery that the B vitamin niacin given to these patients cured the disease led to the complete eradication of this devastating disorder within a few years. Similarly, goiter, due to iodine deficiency, which had affected 40 percent of the schoolchildren in the Midwestern goiter belt, could be cured and further prevented by the simple procedure of fortifying salt with iodine salts.

With the greater knowledge of vitamin and mineral nutrients, U.S. diets in general improved. National and regional nutrition and health surveys indicated that nutrient intakes were generally acceptable, except for some subgroups of the population. However, these same surveys showed that although nutrient

6

intake appeared adequate, the diseases of civilization were on the increase. The prevalance of heart disease, stroke, diabetes, certain cancers, and gastrointestinal disorders alarmingly had increased and epidemiological studies could link these changes to the dietary practices of the population. A reevaluation of our diets was necessary. It was not only important to obtain protein, vitamins, minerals, and energy in sufficient amounts but nonnutrients such as cholesterol or fiber needed to be studied. Furthermore, a great deal of new research had shown that some types of dietary fats and carboyhydrates had positive while others had negative health effects. Of particular interest was the study of the fats in our diets, some of which were significantly associated with heart disease and stroke, and the study of carbohydrates in relation to diabetes and obesity. In a comparatively short period of time, data were obtained that provided a strong impetus for new directions in dietary planning. Although most of the diet-health studies on heart disease, cancer, diabetes, and other diseases have turned out to be extremely complex and scientists still grapple with many unanswered questions, the knowledge gleaned from these studies makes it possible to formulate diets that reduce the risk for these disorders.

New Dietary Goals for Americans

Recognizing the importance of nutrition for good health, the Senate Select Committee on Nutrition and Human Needs in 1977 published the *Dietary Goals for the United States*. This document suggesting dietary changes to reduce chronic disease led to a series of debates. In 1980, the U.S. Department of Agriculture (USDA) and the Department of Health and Human Services (DHHS) jointly published dietary guidelines to help consumers in selecting foods to achieve healthful diets. Following extensive further debates and negotiations with consumer groups, the scientific community, the food industry, and legislators, in 1990 the U.S. Congress passed the Nutrition Labeling and Education Act, which was hailed as one of the most significant legislative acts of the twentieth century. The new regulations addressed primarily three areas:

- the nutrition labeling on foods, which was changed and updated to give the most relevant nutrition information to the consumer,
- the nutrient content of foods,
- and health claims of specific foods.

The final regulations of these changes were implemented by FDA and USDA in 1994.

The new food labels give up-to-date information helpful to the consumer in the planning of healthful diets. The overall objectives of the new labels are to help consumers make healthful food choices, reduce consumer confusion, and give incentives for the food industry to make more healthful foods available to the public (see figure 1).

The second important objective was to develop a *food guide* based on modern nutrition principles, which would allow consumers to make appropriate food choices to promote overall good health. Focusing on the total diet, the food guide aids consumers to select healthful diets that taste good, are satisfying, and can be used throughout life (see figure 2).

The Food Guide Pyramid was developed to help people making appropriate food choices which provide healthful diets.
—**Welch, et al.,** *Nutrition Today* **27(b) (1992): 12–23.**

Based on these exciting national developments, the following chapters highlight the major points important for the consumer. At the end of each chapter, you will find a section on how to apply the information to your specific circumstance and need. You might find that your present diet is in line with the recommendation and is a healthful one. In that case, hearty congratulations! On the other hand, you might find that you could improve your diet in one of several aspects. If this is the case, go for it—it may be the best thing you could do for yourself.

The New Food Label at a Glance *

The new food label will carry an up-to-date, easier-to-use nutrition information guide, to be required on almost all packaged foods (compared to about 60 percent of products up till now). The guide will serve as a key to help in planning a healthy diet.*

Serving sizes are now more consistent across product lines, stated in both household and metric measures, and reflect the amounts people actually eat.

New title signals that the label contains the newly required information.

Calories from fat are now shown on the label to help consumers meet dietary guidelines that recommend people get no more than 30 percent of their calories from fat.

% Daily Value shows how a food fits into the overall daily diet.

The **list of nutrients** covers those most important to the health of today's consumers, most of whom need to worry about getting too much of certain items (fat, for example), rather than too few vitamins or minerals, as in the past.

The label of larger packages must now tell the number of calories per gram of fat, carbohydrate, and protein.

Nutrition Facts

Serving Size ½ cup (114g)
Servings Per Container 4

Amount Per Serving

Calories 90   Calories from Fat 30

                                        % Daily Value*

Total Fat 3g	**5%**
Saturated Fat 0g	**0%**
Cholesterol 0mg	**0%**
Sodium 300mg	**13%**
Total Carbohydrate 13g	**4%**
Dietary Fiber 3g	**12%**
Sugars 3g	
Protein 3g	

Vitamin A	80%	Vitamin C	60%
Calcium	4%	Iron	4%

* Percent Daily Values are based on a 2,000 calorie diet. Your daily values may be higher or lower depending on your calorie needs:

		Calories	2,000	2,500
Total Fat	Less than		65g	80g
Sat Fat	Less than		20g	25g
Cholesterol	Less than		300mg	300mg
Sodium	Less than		2,400mg	2,400mg
Total Carbohydrate			300g	375g
Fiber			25g	30g

Calories per gram:
Fat 9 • Carbohydrate 4 • Protein 4

Daily Values are also something new. Some are maximums, as with fat (65 grams or less); others are minimums, as with carbohydrate (300 grams or more). The daily values for a 2,000- and 2,500-calorie diet must be listed on the label of larger packages. Individuals should adjust the values to fit their own calorie intake.

* This label is only a sample. Exact specifications are in the final rules.
Source: Food and Drug Administration 1993

Figure 1

*Danielle Shor and Charles Edwards, "USDA's Role: Nutrition Labeling of Meat and Poultry Products," *Nutrition Today* 28 (5) 1993 (reprinted by permission).

The Food Pyramid

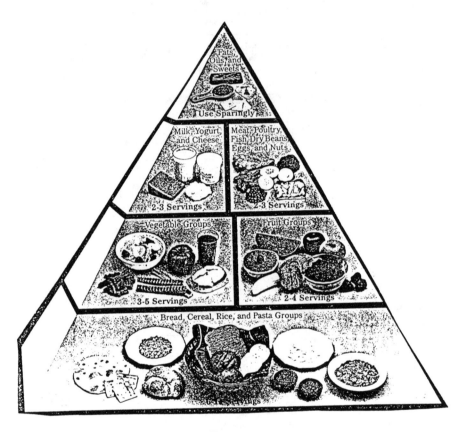

Figure 2

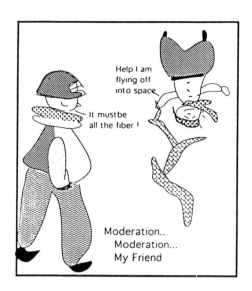

Chapter II
Healthful Diets Is the Theme

We can answer the question, What is a healthful diet? on several levels. We can evaluate our diets to decide whether or not we are on the right track by using comparatively simple criteria. These are *variety, balance,* and *moderation.* This triad has been consciously or unconsciously practiced by many peoples throughout human history. Today these criteria have taken on a new meaning because of the scientific evidence that supports them.

Variety Is Vogue

The reason that we should eat a variety of foods is that *no single food provides the nutrients and calories children and adults need.* A diet that includes a variety of foods is more likely to provide us with all the essential nutrients our bodies require.

We start life with nourishment from one food—human milk or sometimes from milk-based formulas patterned on human milk. For the first few months of life, human milk is an ideal food because the nutrients are adequate, easily digestible, and absorbable, and furthermore provide immune bodies that protect the infant from infectious disease. During the first few months of life, the infant also uses nutrients that had been stored during intrauterine life in its liver. Milk, for example, is a poor source of iron; the newborn uses iron stored in its liver for blood formation. The immature gut of the newborn infant precludes the eating of foods that the adult can chew and digest.

Weaning the infant from a complete milk diet starts the slow process of learning to eat a variety of foods. Weaning can be a slow or a more rapid process during which foods other than milk are introduced. By approximately four to five months of life, human milk needs to be supplemented with extra food to provide more protein and calories as well as iron for adequate continued growth and development. Toward the end of the second year, the young child has learned to eat a variety of foods and usually can eat foods of different tastes, flavors, textures, and consistency.

Therefore a critical period to introduce a variety of foods is during the latter part of infancy. A new food should be given, a little only, when the child is hungry. Wait a few days to see whether the child gets a reaction to the food before giving more. Don't introduce new foods when the child does not feel well and do not force a child to eat. Even at the age of one or two, children imitate their parents; therefore parents need to be role models. Rarely will a child come to like a food parents dislike. Acquiring the habit of eating a variety of foods is a learning process and an important lesson each child needs to learn.

By twelve months a baby should be feeding him/herself almost entirely. The next big step for the child involves learning when to eat (and when not to eat), what manners are, and how to imitate adults. Over the next five to six years children will learn how to eat like other people by modeling their behavior on adults, but this learning comes gradually.
—Interview with T. Berry Brazelton, M.D., *Journal of the American Dietetic Association* (1993): 1385–88. Copyright The American Dietetic Association. Reprinted by permission from Journal of The American Dietetic Association, Vol. 93.

Another critical period in establishing adult food habits is during adolescence. Peer pressure affects the food selection of children and young adults. There is no guarantee that children can withstand it completely. Parents must make sure that the adolescent at least has one good meal per day. Offer plenty of fruits, whole-grain cereals, low-fat milk instead of cakes and chips and soft drinks. Children who have been used to eating varied and nutritious foods may wander to experience junk foods but usually get tired of them and return to what they have been used to.

By the early twenties, people's food habits usually are firmly established. Reeducation for consumption of a variety of foods and to change food likes and dislikes after this time is often problematic, especially when food is used as the main pleasure giver in a person's life. Changing a diet is possible, especially if the changes make a person feel better, but often is difficult, and time-consuming reeducation efforts are required.

To change an undesirable trait, you must zero in on exactly what it is you need to change. A "list technique" will help. All you need is a pencil and paper. And honesty.

The Balancing Act

A second criterion used to evaluate and plan diets is *balance*. For years people have talked about eating balanced diets, but what does it really mean? Even if we eat daily a variety of foods, we can go wrong if their proportions are unfavorable. Imagine for a minute a three-ounce hamburger and half a teaspoon of mustard. You would still consume the same two foods if you were to have three ounces of mustard and half a teaspoon of hamburger! But what an unpalatable combination! While proportionality is easy to grasp when taste is concerned, balance usually means something less obvious. Balance or proportionality means that the essential nutrients together with energy need to be consumed in certain proportions. If, for example, you increase your energy need by starting a vigorous exercise program, the need for several B vitamins increases also. Another example is the intake of polyunsaturated oils, which require proportionately more dietary vitamin E. Nutrients are utilized in the body according to specific proportions. In general, nutrients are provided in acceptable proportions from diets that include a variety of wholesome foods. Imbalance occurs when whole food groups such as dairy products, vegetables, or fruits are omitted, when too many refined foods are eaten, or when vitamin and mineral supplements are consumed in excess. Caloric imbalances are common and the consumption of foods with high proportions of total and saturated fats has been shown to be detrimental to heatlh.

14

Despite billions of dollars spent by consumers each year on weight-loss pills, potions, and programs, at least 26 percent of the total population in this country is overweight and at any one particular time about 65 million Americans report they are dieting.

A growing body of evidence demonstrates that people are overweight for many different reasons—social, genetic, dietary, metabolic, and psychological. A common comment made by people losing weight is that they decrease their total calories slightly together with a sharp reduction in fat intake.

—P. Foreyt, *Journal of the American Dietetic Association* (1992): Insert 1–6. Copyright The American Dietetic Association. Reprinted by permission from JOURNAL OF THE AMERICAN DIETETIC ASSOCIATION, Vol. 92.

A new kind of balance appreciated only quite recently is that one food can interfere with the nutrient absorption of another. For example, high-fiber diets may decrease the gastrointestinal absorption of some trace minerals. The high phosphate content of milk interferes with iron absorption. Conversely, the vitamin C in orange juice and other foods helps the body to absorb iron from some foods. The concept of balance related to the availability of nutrients from food mixtures is a difficult one, and a great deal is not yet sufficiently researched. When people limit the amount they eat in order to lose weight, it is especially important that all nutrients in their food be available to be used to the fullest extent possible.

Use Moderation

You can eat a varied diet with the foods in perfect balance and yet you may have a problem if you eat too much or too little. Moderation in eating prevents obesity and several other diseases. Moderation also helps in the prevention of eating too little, which can lead to starvation and malnutrition as it occurs in anorexia nervosa. As with exercise and sleep, we need to find the golden mean for our food intake. What is moderate may vary from person to person and is sometimes difficult to arrive at. Knowledge of acceptable portion sizes will help in the planning of moderate food intakes. Moderation in food intake is also a guide in the prevention of "binging" on specific foods. A person who "binges" needs to find out the conditions that set off this behavior. In addition to medical treatment, planning alternative food strategies is exceedingly important. The easy availability of junk food in the house may encourage "binging," but the substitution of fruits and wholesome cereals may lessen such frantic behavior.

Variety, balance, and moderation of your food intake are the three pillars that support good nutrition. Any one of them, if inadequate, will shake the foundation of your health and well-being. Unfortunately, many of us find out too late that not all is well. After the first heart attack or stroke, or when we have become obese, it may be all too late. In the long run, preventing traveling down the path of nutritional ignorance is less painful, less expensive, and can be infinitely more enjoyable. The guideposts of dietary variety, balance, and moderation are a helpful first step in planning diets for long-term health. They are also tools for a quick self-evaluation whether you are on the right track. Changing living arrangements almost always affects one's diet and the criteria of variety, balance, and moderation will be helpful guides to reestablish and continue a healthful lifestyle.

Every evaluation of a person's nutritional adequacy must start with an assessment of what a person eats. Food intakes change from day to day, but most people follow established predictable patterns. The first concern and starting point for the evaluation of your food behaviors therefore is to document what you usually eat. Ideally you should look at your food intake over several days or a whole week to include the weekend. By comparing your daily food intake with standards, you may find that your usual diet is adequate. Or you may find that you need to change your diet in one or several aspects. At the end of this section, an outline is given for the initial part of your evaluation. With each further section, a new area of nutrition will be added to conclude evaluation and diet planning as a twelve-step program taken on consecutive days or spread over a period of time.

16

Step One: Food Behaviors Can Tell You a Lot

If anybody offers you advice on diet without taking stock of your present diet, be critical. Some very strange food habits are based on such lopsided advice. Fred, for example, was advised to use low-fat milk to cut down on milk fat. He religiously used low-fat milk in his diet but ate a pint of ice cream every day! Many other such examples could be cited. To know if your diet is acceptable, you must start looking at your total diet first.

To evaluate your own diet and to make improvements, if necessary, take a few minutes every day over the next twelve days and look at your diet critically. The exercises at the end of each chapter will help you to evaluate your dietary practices. You may find your diet is adequate, or you may find you need to improve one or several areas of your diet.

First you need to document what your present diet looks like. Preferably, we should look at food intake over several days. But selecting a typical day, let's just look at food eaten during this one day. Write down all foods eaten at meals and snacks and any drinks you have consumed. Just record everything you have put into your mouth. If you easily forget, make notes as you go through the day. It is surprising how automatic eating gets and this makes it more difficult to remember what you have eaten. Enter all types of food and the time of the meal or snack in the attached daily food intake form. Also try to evaluate the portions of each food (for example, six ounces of orange juice, a slice of whole wheat bread, etc.) This will not be very accurate. Don't worry about perfect accuracy in amounts. Fill out the four columns in the attached form (see page 18) to represent your food intake as closely as you can. Please, no cheating! Keep the food intake record—we all need it as we go along—and look at different aspects of your diet.

For now, answer just a few questions related to your food behaviors:

1. How many meals did you eat per day?
2. Did you eat breakfast or did you skip it?
3. How often do you snack per day?

4. From cursory inspection do you think your food intake is well spaced throughout the day or are you heavily favoring one specific meal?
5. How many meals or snacks prepared outside the home did you eat?
6. Did you at any time of the day feel hungry?
7. Do you feel your food intake is at the present time adequate or should it be improved? (Keep your one-day food intake. We will use it again.)

The answers will tell you something about your meal plan and the distribution of food during the day. Are you a meal eater, a nibbler, or a snacker? Do you rely on somebody else for your meals? What do you perceive as problems with your diet? Make a list of the points that come to your mind, and as we go along, we will address the issues that shape acceptable dietary practices. Keep your food intake list, and if you wish, write down several other daily intakes. We will process them further in subsequent sections.

Your Food Intake for One Day (Date)

Time	Type of Food Eaten	Quantity of Food	Food Group

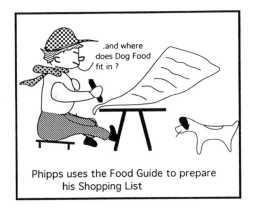

.and where does Dog Food fit in ?

Phipps uses the Food Guide to prepare his Shopping List

Chapter III
Food Savvy

To select nutritious diets, knowledge of foods is a must. Supermarkets and specialty stores offer a confusing selection of basic foods, innumerable prepared items, and even fully prepared meals. Foods attractively packaged tempt the shopper, and persuasive ads create the desire to buy. This is a very different situation from that of our grandmothers who baked their own bread, grew their own vegetables, and kept small and large livestock for eggs, milk, and meat. While they largely had to rely on their own, often limited resources of food, we today have a virtually limitless choice of foods all year round.

With so many foods available at all times, are we choosing wisely? Selecting foods is a complex task. Economics, familiarity with particular foods, availability, food-likes and dislikes all play a part. And what about nutritional adequacy and health issues? More than at any other time, health considerations have come to the forefront. Old entrenched ideas are questioned, and the advances in nutrition research provide guidance in the selection of healthful diets. While the "ideal diet" has proved elusive, we have ample evidence that some nutritional practices are detrimental while others are beneficial. We have learned that diets are no cure-alls, but if chosen well can give us stamina, well-being and may be instrumental in preventing chronic disease.

Foods: Bearers of Nutrients

Only a small number of the myriad plants and animals in nature are used as food for human consumption. Yet even this small percentage is large enough to provide the many foods grown and sold around the world. The plants and animals acceptable as foods share several commonalities. As carriers of nutrients and calories, they satisfy our nutritional needs and have acceptable taste and flavor qualities. Foods must also be free from harmful substances, such as poisons or undesirable microbial contamination.

However, we find that foods differ vastly in their nutrient composition. Each food is unique and no food provides exactly the same type and amount of nutrients as the next. Some foods are practically devoid of one or several nutrients, while others are rich sources. For example, an orange that has no fat is rich in vitamin C, meat is a good source of iron but poor in calcium. Even one specific food may vary in one or several nutrients, depending on conditions of growth, storage, refining, and other environmental factors.

Measuring the nutrient content of foods has been a long and arduous endeavor and is still continuing. While the exact nutrient composition for some foods is still problematic, most commonly used foods are remarkably well studied and their protein, vitamin, mineral, and calorie content is well known. Based on these data, we classify foods into six groups of similar nutrient strengths and weaknesses. Such a grouping, although somewhat artificial, makes meal planning and evaluation of nutrient adequacy less cumbersome. Several food group models have been suggested and tried in the past. The latest model using six food groups is especially useful since it allows food planning for nutrient adequate diets coupled with the long-term prevention of chronic disease. A brief outline of this particular food grouping is given in the following section.

Goals of the New Food Group Guide

1. To promote overall health
2. They are based on up-to-date research
3. They focus on the total diet
4. They are useful for the public
5. They meet nutritional goals in a realistic manner
6. They are practical

—S. Welsh, et al., Development of the Food Guide Pyramid, *Nutrition Today* 27(6) 1992: 12–23.

Food Grouping for Simplicity

The *GRAIN / BREAD / CEREAL GROUP* provides the largest contribution to our energy needs. Food energy, measured in calories, is the first important need of our body. Without energy all other nutrients cannot work. Without fuel, a car, a heater, a steam engine will not work. We get our needed fuel from food. Without it we survive for a while by burning our own flesh, but after several days of starvation, our body machinery slowly begins to shut down.

In addition to the energy content, grain products provide a number of nutrients in significant amounts. Whole grains are rich in fiber, several B vitamins, and several trace minerals. Milling reduces the nutrient content and fiber, but the energy in finely milled white flour is not affected. Refined cereals, breads, and pasta are generally lower in nutrients than whole grain products. Fortification to produce "enriched" products adds back only some of the nutrients that had been removed during refining. Many cereals are fortified and contain higher amounts of vitamins and minerals than are present in the original grain product. These additions are listed on the labels of cereal boxes.

Grains are the staple foods of peoples around the world. Rice in Japan and China, corn in Central America, wheat in the United States and Europe have been traditional foods for centuries. Modern food processing has modified the basic staples and today innumerable types of cereals, breads, pastas are manufactured and sold not only in the United States but around the globe. It is not always easy to recognize the ingredients of such foods, and reading nutrition labels has become an indispensable tool to get information about a food. Taste, flavor, and consistency of grain/bread/cereal foods can vary considerably. Originally the grains provided bland calorie-containing foods, which were eaten with a variety of flavorful side dishes, such as spicy Mexican peppers or soy products with rice to make flavorful combinations and the staples more palatable.

Wheat, corn, oats, barley, rice, rye, and millet are staple foods around the globe. They are consumed as grains, cereals, breads, pasta and are ingredients in many mixed foods and should provide us with the major portion of our energy needs.

Today modern supermarkets provide us with almost limitless possibilities of foods from the grain group to satisfy every taste and preference. Two points are of vital importance here. Inclusion of some high-fiber products is vital. Each one of us needs to find our own level of fiber we can tolerate. Too much may give you diarrhea and sleepless nights; too little may result in unpleasant constipation. Find the level of fiber good for you. Your optimum may be different from anybody else's. Together with fiber-rich foods, we need to drink fluid—water, juice, coffee, tea—since fiber eaten alone may also lead to constipation.

The second point in selecting servings from the grain/bread/cereal group is to keep sugar, syrups, and other high-calorie sweetners down to a minimum. Sugar is added to many foods, sometimes hidden, at other times obvious. For centuries sugar has been used as a sweetening agent and to preserve foods. We like sweet-tasting foods; they give us pleasure and gratification. Sugars provide practically the same amount of energy as starch (weight for weight). However, our body works better with starch than sugars. Sugars are absorbed into our bloodstream very rapidly and can contribute to diabetes in sensitive people. Table sugar (sucrose) is a highly refined product, so is honey. Both are desirable sweetening agents. Their use as a significant energy source on the other hand is detrimental because sugar and honey provide only empty calories.

For healthful diets, grain and grain products should provide our body with at least half the energy we require. Some high-fiber products should be selected daily. Cereals and other grain products with too much sugar should be used sparingly. Highly refined products, which have lost some or all of their nutrients, should be used sparingly.

The *VEGETABLE GROUP* and the *FRUIT GROUP* are sometimes discussed together because of similar nutrient strength and weakness. Both groups offer an almost unlimited number of foods all year round. Some fruits and vegetables are only available in season and thrifty shoppers will look for products in season. Half a cup of broccoli, carrots, peas, or an apple, half a banana, a glass of orange juice would be considered one serving. The daily recommendation is to include at least three servings from the vegetable and two servings from the fruit group.

Variety is again essential, and selection should vary. It's important to include a good source of vitamin C daily, such as citrus fruit, green pepper, or broccoli. Cooking will destroy some of the vitamin C and other vitamins, so vegetables should be cooked as briefly as possible and with little cooking water. Vitamin C will help in the absorption of dietary iron and has a possible role in cancer prevention. A daily source of one yellow or green vegetable will provide beta-carotene; dark green leafy vegetables provide folic acid, vitamin K, and magnesium. Furthermore, vegetables and fruits are excellent sources of fiber. Vegetables can be used raw, in salads, and cooked in many different ways, such as in stews and soups, mixed or singly. Fruits are eaten raw or cooked, or as juices. The choices are almost limitless.

Each fruit and vegetable is a storehouse of antioxidants, prooxidants, carcinogens, and antimutagens, with the balance perhaps in favor of the anticarcinogens in a diet based on moderation, variety, and balance.
   —Herbert Victor, M.D., J.D., "Viewpoint. Does mega-C do more good than harm, or more harm than good?" *Nutrition Today* 28(1) (1993): 28–32.

Food items from the *MILK/DAIRY GROUP* need to be carefully selected especially to satisfy proportionality in your diet. Milk, yogurt, and other milk products (except butter and cream) are major sources of dietary calcium, vitamin D, and the B vitamin riboflavin in addition to protein. We want to encourage sufficient calcium intake for everybody throughout life. The highest daily calcium amounts are required by teenage boys and girls and during pregnancy and lactation to achieve good bone growth. To retard bone loss due to osteoporosis, elderly women may require more than two cups of milk per day. Two cups of milk per day, or yogurt, will provide approximately 600 mg of calcium per day. Cottage or other cheeses can be substituted for some milk.

One drawback of foods from the milk group is the milk fat, of which the most concentrated form is butter and cream. Fat from cow's milk is a highly saturated fat, the type of fat that encourages heart disease. The first deposits of fatty material (cholesterol and fats) in the arteries of people may already start as early as the childhood years. Although the progress of atherosclerosis in early adulthood is usually insidiously slow, eventually a heart attack or stroke may occur. In a preventive effort to decrease the risk of atherosclerosis, dairy products low in fat should be selected.

In the United States, in addition to whole milk and whole-milk dairy products, several fat-modified milks, yogurts, cottage, ricotta, and other cheeses are on the market (skim, 1 percent fat, 2 percent fat). Adults on varied diets do usually well if they select a product of their liking with reduced fat content. Individuals who have one or several family members suffering from premature heart disease (in particular, a parent with premature heart disease and atherosclerosis) should start to reduce dairy fat during childhood (after two years of age) in a preventive effort. Lacto-vegetarians who rely heavily on the dairy group as a protein source are another group of people who may obtain too much milkfat in their diets. The dairy product with highest saturated fat content is butter. Use it sparingly, if at all. Substituting vegetable oil or soft margarine for some of the butter will add less saturated fat to your diet, but there is still the controversial question of the trans-fatty acids in partially hydrogenated margarine, which may be as atherogenic as butter. Weight for weight the calories in margarine are the same as in butter.

Although milk and dairy products are excellent foods providing several necessary nutrients, the scientific data show overwhelmingly that the saturated fat from dairy (and other foods) encourages atherosclerosis. Since today the separation of milk fat from milk is an easy process, dairy products with lower fat content are sold widely, and people can take advantage of these superior nutritious foods that by their reduced fat content are made into highly healthful food items.

Dr. Willett, in his article on "Diet and Health: What should you eat?" which appeared in *Science* 264 (1994): 532–537, suggests that different saturated fats influence blood cholesterol (LDL levels) differently. Butter and dairy fats high in myristic acid strongly increase blood cholesterol while beef fat has a lesser (but still significant) effect. (Abstracted with permission from *Science* 264 [1994]. Copyright 1994 American Association for the Advancement of Science.)

The *MEAT/POULTRY/FISH/LEGUMES/EGG GROUP* contains a diverse selection of animal foods including eggs but also vegetable products such as dry soybean flour, beans, peas, and lentils. They are listed together because they are excellent protein sources. Again variety and moderation are the key when selecting foods from this group. In addition to protein, these foods provide other constituents; some of these are desirable, others may be harmful. Egg is a good protein source but also provides cholesterol. Red meat provides iron but is a source of fat, undesirable in relation to atherosclerosis. Ocean fish is rich in essential fatty acids, which are beneficial in the prevention of disease. Legumes contain carbohydrates, including fiber, in addition to protein.

In the past, diets in the United States have been planned with meat as the main dish of a meal and vegetables, potatoes, corn, rice, and pasta as side dishes. We need to reeducate ourselves and use vegetables, salads, pasta, etc., as main dishes, with small portions of meat on the side. The fat in meats—visible and invisible—and the cholesterol in eggs are the major reasons why we need to select foods from this group sparingly. Substitute fish, chicken, or legumes for some of the meat. Half a cup of baked beans, lentils, or cooked dry peas are equivalent to the protein of one ounce of lean meat (see table 1).

26

Table 1

Choose Lean Beef from the Skinniest Six

	Cals	Per 3 oz* Total Fat	Saturated Fat
Top Round	169	4.2 grams	1.5 grams
Top Loin	168	7.1 grams	2.7 grams
Eye of the Round	141	4.0 grams	1.5 grams
Sirloin	162	5.8 grams	2.2 grams
Tenderloin	185	8.1 grams	3.0 grams
Round Tip	149	5.0 grams	1.8 grams

*fat trimmed off
USDA Handbook 8–13, 1990

FATS / OIL / SUGAR / ALCOHOL / SALT are lumped together even though they are very different in their caloric content and also in how the body handles them. Salt does not quite fit into this group since it does not provide calories. Highly salted foods should be limited because of their relationship with hypertension (see mineral section). Fats, oils, sugar, and alcohol all provide empty calories. An exception are the oils that contain polyunsaturated fats and some vitamin E and K.

Fats and oils give a pleasant taste to many foods and are used in many cooking recipes, but we must remember that all fats and oils are very high calorie sources. Weight for weight they provide more than twice the calories in carbohydrates and proteins. Many foods contain naturally high amounts of fats or oils, such as olives and avocados, fatty meats, skin of chicken, and nuts. Foods to which fat has been added during processing are also high in fats, such as tuna packed in oil, or mayonnaise. Food products high in fat and oils need to be selected carefully in terms of *total fat content* and the *type of fat* they provide. Label reading is paramount. Unfortunately, not all foods are labeled to indicate their total amount of fat and the type of fat they contain.

Learning to read food labels will help you to learn about foods.

Sugar provides empty calories and is part of a host of other products like cakes, pies, cookies, sweetened cereals, canned fruits, jams, jellies, ice creams, chocolate, and candies. It is hidden in such products as tomato paste, soft drinks, and sweets. Sugar can be used to great advantage as a flavoring agent but needs to be used sparingly. Fats and sugar provide empty calories; they should never provide the major portion of your daily energy need.

Step Two: How Does Your Diet Rate?

To evaluate your own diet for variety and balance, go back to your Food Intake Record prepared during "Step One" and assign each food you have eaten to the appropriate food group. If you are not sure to which group a food belongs, consult the food list at the end of this exercise. If you have eaten a mixed dish like pizza, for example, you need to list it under several groups, such as the bread/grain (crust), the milk/dairy group (cheese), and the vegetable group (tomato). List sugar, honey, sweets, butter, oils, other fats, and alcohol in the last group. When completed, add up the total number of servings for each group and answer the following questions:

1. Have you selected foods from the cereal, vegetable, fruit, milk, and meat group?
2. Have you omitted foods from one food group completely?
3. Are foods from one or two groups overrepresented?
4. Is one favorite food eaten in excess?
5. How many alcoholic beverages did you consume?
6. Now compare your food intake with the recommendation below:

28

Table 2

Recommended Food Intake

Food Group	Grain	Vegetable	Fruit	Milk	Meat	FSA*
Recommended no. of servings	6	3	2	2	3	
Your servings	( )	( )	( )	( )	( )	( )

*Foods from the fat/sugar/alcohol group should be low.

To check your diet for variety, compare whether you get the recommended servings from each of the five groups. Further check whether you eat a variety of foods from each group. If you have several items in the FSA (fat/sugar/alcohol) group, this should be of concern to you. If you have problems eating the recommended servings from the major food groups, think of ways to improve your diet.

Comments (Step One and Two Exercise)

Whether we eat acceptable diets or whether we need to make changes cannot be determined without looking critically at our daily food intake. A baseline of our food intake will tell us what changes need to be made. The one-day example you have just finished is a paradigm for a quick review of how varied your diet is, whether you eat foods from all the recommended food groups, or whether your diet relies heavily on empty calories from the FSA group. Meal and snack spacing during the day also was noted. If you find odd meal spacing, glaring omissions, or unusual food patterns, follow your diet for several days, preferably a whole week. This will give you a better baseline from which to start to improve your diet.

Grains/Bread/Cereal/Pasta/Starch Group

Whole grains all kinds
Breads, all kinds
    White
    Whole grain
Buns and rolls, all kinds
Pita bread
    White
    Whole grain
Pumpernickel, rye
Tortilla
Corn breads
Muffins, all kinds
    Bran
    Fruit
Cereals
    Whole grain
    Unsweetened
    Sweetened

Wheat germ
Pasta, all kinds
Rice, white and brown
Crackers, all kinds
    White
    Whole grain
Pancakes
Waffles

Legumes
    Lentils, peas
    Baked beans

Starchy vegetables
    Potato, all kinds
    Corn, cob or cereals
    Yams, sweet potatoes
    Winter squash

Vegetable Group

Asparagus
Artichoke
Bean sprouts
Broccoli
Brussels sprouts
Cabbage, all kinds
Carrots
Cauliflower
Eggplant
Peppers, all kinds
Greens
    Beets
    Chard
    Collards

Dandelion
Kale
Mustard
Spinach
Turnip
Kohlrabi
Leeks
Mushrooms
Okra
Onion
Peas
Rutabaga
Sauerkraut
String beans, all kinds

Squash, all kinds
Turnip
Water chestnuts
Wax beans

Zucchini
Vegetable juices
    Tomato
    Mixed

Fruit Group

Apple
Applesauce, unsweetened
Apricots, fresh, dried, canned
Banana
Berries, fresh
    Blackberries
    Blueberries
    Gooseberries
    Loganberries
    Raspberries
    Strawberries
Cherries fresh, canned
Dates
Figs, fresh, dried
Fruit cocktail
Grapefruit, fresh, juice
Grapes
Kiwi
Mango

Melon, all kinds
    Cantaloupe
    Honeydew
    Watermelon
Nectarine
Orange, fresh, juice
Papaya
Peach, fresh, canned
Pear, fresh, canned
Persimmons
Pineapple, fresh, canned
Plums
Pomegranate
Prunes
Raisins
Tangerine
All fruit juices
Orange, grapefruit, apple,
Cranberry, apricot, cider, etc.

Milk/Dairy Group

Milk and yogurt
    Fat-free
    1% fat
    2% fat
    4% fat (whole milk)
Buttermilk, acidophilus
Soy milk

Cheeses, fat-controlled
    Cottage, fat-free
    1%, 2%, 4% fat
    Ricotta fat-free
    1%, 2%, 4% fat
Cheeses, other, all kinds

Mozzarella, Parmesan,
   Camembert,
Edam, Jarlsberg,
   Liederkranz,

Swiss, Feta, Cheddar,
   Gruyere, Gorgonzola,
Munster, Gouda,
   American processed

Meat/Protein Group

Select lean items, well trimmed of fat, cook without added fat, skim fat off stews

Beef
Pork
Lamb/mutton
Veal
Poultry
   Chicken
   Turkey
Fish, all kinds
Game
   Rabbit
   Venison

Legumes
   Baked beans, no pork
   Lentils
   Dried peas
Items high in cholesterol
   Liver
   Sweetbreads
   Eggs
Items high in fat and salt
   Cold cuts and sausages
   Hot dogs, ham, and bacon

High Fat/High Sugar/High Salt/and Alcohol Group

This group includes a hodgepodge of items that can be added to a good diet **but which should not replace nutritious food items.** Most of the items in this group, except some of the high-salt foods such as vegetable pickles, are high in calories. Common representatives of this group are:

Solid fats. These include products such as lard, beef fat, chicken fat, vegetable shortening, butter, coconut fat, tropical seed fats, margarine. Products to which fats have been added, such as chips, french fries, and deep-fried foods.

32

Processed meats: Cold cuts, hot dogs, sausages often are not defined as far as their total fat, type of fat, and their salt content. Individuals who start putting together a basic diet should go slow with foods of this type. Occasional inclusion of a processed meat should be in moderate quantities.

Oils. These are also high in calories, but some is necessary daily to provide the polyunsaturated fats. Polyunsaturated fats can be obtained from salad dressings and mayonnaise, although the latter also contains egg and therefore cholesterol.

Sugar. This is found in foods such as table sugar, syrups, honey, and candies, sweets and chocolates of all kinds. Foods with high sugar content include rich cakes, cookies, desserts, and cereals high in sugar (read labels).

Ice creams. All kinds are high in sugar and fat.

Cream. Sweet and sour cream, half and half are all high-calorie items with high amounts of saturated fats.

Soft drinks. Coca Cola, Mountain Dew, orange soda, Dr. Pepper-type soda, Pepsi Cola, 7UP, and others contain per 12 fluid ozs. between 144 and 184 Cal equivalent to seven and eight heaped teaspoons full of table sugar.

Processed foods. If composition is unknown, we cannot evaluate calories, sugar, fat content, and the type of fat. If contents are listed for a product, the major ingredient is listed first.

Alcohol. Beer, wine, liquors provide empty calories.

Prepared meals. Prepared whole meals can be helpful for the busy person who has little time to cook or who cannot cook.

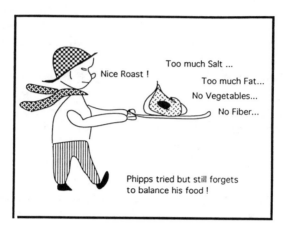

Chapter IV
Know the Basics

Your diet must provide the nutrients and calories you need, be tasty, satisfying, and sustain your health on a long-term basis. It furthermore must fit your pocketbook and your time available for food preparation. Children's diets in addition need to provide nutrients for optimum growth and development.

These requirements are a tall order. To accomplish them, you need to select and prepare your diet thoughtfully. It is not sufficient to cook a good meal. Meals are an important part of our daily diet, but everything that enters our mouth—snacks, between-meal goodies, late-night treats, alcoholic and nonalcoholic beverages—is part of a person's daily intake. We can only judge whether our diet is varied, balanced, and moderate if we take into account the whole day's food intake, absolutely everything we have consumed.

The first step toward *variety, balance, and moderation* in our daily diet is achieved by:

1. Eating daily foods from the cereal, vegetable, fruit, dairy, and meat groups.
2. Learning the numbers and appropriate portion sizes for food items in the five food groups.
3. Incorporating the portions of the selected foods into daily menus that are mouth-watering and pleasing.

By using these simple criteria, we can easily recogize glaring dietary problems, such as omitting all dairy foods, or eating a decidely imbalanced diet. The plan is flexible to accommodate individual preferences, variations in ethnic foods, and the likelihood of possible nutrient deficiency is at a minimum. Such a plan allows us to make calorie adjustments for specific conditions, such as weight reduction, diets for athletes, pregnant women, and the elderly.

Eating a variety of foods already achieves a great deal toward a healthful diet, but it is a first step only. It provides a framework for the selection of foods. As we will see in a later section, greater familiarity with this process allows us to fine-tune our diets within this framework. For the final adjustment, we need to know something about the composition of foods, their similarities and differences. Some of these differences are critical for our health.

Meal Eating versus Nibbling

It is possible to eat one's daily food in just one meal. There are people who can eat a lot in one session and then wait twenty-four hours for the next meal. But such folks are rare. Most people in the United States eat the traditional three meals per day, with one or several snacks in between meals. In recent years two meals per day—brunch and dinner—have become popular, especially for young women who are concerned about getting obese. Then there are individuals who snack throughout the day and have no regular meals at all. Although eating patterns vary widely, selecting a variety of foods from the basic food groups is vitally important and is applicable to whatever eating patterns a person follows.

Whether to snack or to follow a fixed meal pattern depends on preference and sometimes on one's lifestyle. From animal studies we know that one large meal per day encourages fat deposition. Regularity in eating has been associated with well-being and sustained performance throughout the day. Regular meals also prevent overeating at one meal and the resulting discomfort of eating a large meal. With the rapidly increasing tendency to eat more meals outside the home, we need to be concerned about the nutritional value of such food and to consider meals and snacks eaten away from home as a part of our daily diet.

Know Your Serving Size

As important as the types of food we choose is their amounts. The quantification of food is usually done by the serving size, which is simply the amount of a food usually consumed by the majority of people. However, the perception of a serving size differs from person to person, and sometimes varies a lot. A hungry person may select a much larger serving size than the average, while a person who does not like a particular food will select a small portion. Because of these factors, nutritionists have introduced standard servings for most foods. With a little practice, serving sizes or standard portions can be learned. Such portions are defined by their weight, or volume, or size. In food composition tables, nutrient values and calories are usually given for standard serving sizes (calories of a slice of bread, or grams of protein per cup of milk, for example). The portion size of foods is a convenient unit that allows us to plan diets and to calculate the caloric and nutrient content of diets. If we start with standard serving sizes, we can also increase or decrease the number of the serving size, depending on a person's need. An athlete in training, for example, would increase the number of servings from the cereal group, while a person on a weight-reduction diet would decrease the number and the size of servings of a calorie-rich food (see table 3).

The Food Guide in Action

Table 3

How Much Is One Serving?

Food Group	Serving Sizes
Grain/rice/pasta	1 slice of bread
	1/2 hamburger roll, bagel, muffin
	1/2 cup rice, pasta, cooked cereal
	3–4 plain crackers
Vegetable	1/2 cup chopped raw or cooked
	1 cup leafy raw vegetables
	3/4 cup vegetable juice
Fruits	1 medium whole fruit or melon wedge
	1/2 cup canned or chopped fruit
	1/4 cup dried fruit
	6 oz fruit juice
Milk	1 cup milk or yogurt
	1 1/2 oz cheese
	2 oz processed cheese
Meat	1 oz well-trimmed meat, poultry, fish
	1/2 cup baked beans, lentils, peas
	1 egg, 2 tablespoons peanut butter all count as 1 oz meat
Fat/oil/sugar/alcohol	limit

In the following we walk leisurely through the planning of your diet. It may seem cumbersome at first, but if you have done this once, you get the idea about what's important and with practice it will take almost no time at all. Let's assume you want to plan your own diet for one day. Let's further assume that you are a fairly inactive person. The step you would take is to select the recommended servings from the five food groups (consult the food pyramid). Your diet would include at a minimum the following servings:

Food Group	Servings
Grain/cereal/bread	6
Vegetables	3
Fruits	2
Milk/dairy	2–3
Meat/and meat substitutes	5

The next step would identify the actual foods and their serving sizes as the following diet for one day shows.

6 servings from the grain group:	Servings
2 slices of bread	2
1/2 cup cereal	1
1 cup rice or pasta	2
4 small crackers	1

3 servings from the vegetable group:	
1/2 cup broccoli	1
1/2 cup mixed salad	1
1/2 cup carrots	1

<u>2 to 3 servings of fruits:</u>

6 oz orange juice	1
1 medium apple	1
1/2 banana	1

<u>2 to 3 servings from the milk group:</u>

1 cup milk low fat	1
1 cup yogurt low fat	1
3/4 oz of cheese	0.5

<u>5 servings from the meat group:</u>

3 oz lean meat, poultry, or fish	3
1/2 cup cooked legumes	1
1 egg	1

The next step is to distribute these foods throughout the day in a meal plan of your preference. The following is an example of a conventional three-meal plan with a late evening snack.

Breakfast

Cereal, 1/2 cup	1 grain
milk, 1/2 cup 1% fat	1/2 milk
orange juice, 6 oz	1 fruit
coffee, black	

Lunch

chicken breast, 3 oz	3 meat
2 slices of whole-wheat bread	2 grain
lettuce, 1/2 cup	1 vegetable
1/2 a banana	1 fruit
beverage	

Supper

rice, 1 cup	2 grain
broccoli, 1/2 cup	1 vegetable
carrots, 1/2 cup	1 vegetable
cooked dry beans, 1/2 cup	1 meat substitute
egg	1 meat substitute
1 apple	1 fruit
yogurt, 1 cup	1 milk

Late night snack

4 crackers	1 grain
cheese, 1.5 oz	1 milk

Total servings for one day: grain 6; vegetable 3; fruits 3; milk 2.5; meat 5.

Note that this diet plan does not contain any foods classified in the fat/oil/sugar group. If we calculate the nutrients and calories of this diet, we find that this is a very low-calorie diet, which provides sufficient protein, vitamins, and minerals. The addition of salad dressing, a pat of butter, and a little cooking oil will increase the calories in this diet.

The above example is a demonstration of how to plan a day's menu for variety, balance, and proportionality. It may seem daunting at first glance, but if you have worked through it once or twice, you get the idea. After consciously planning a good diet for a period, doing it becomes routine and almost second nature. The crux is to select servings from the various food groups and put them together in a way to make satisfying meals. There is a lot of leeway to be creative. The plan also enables you to be economical yet make nutritious and tasty meals. Each food group has an extraordinary number of foods to choose from to suit every taste and preference.

Table 4

Servings Measured in Hand-Size Equivalents

A thumb	=	1 ounce of cheese
A thumb tip	=	1 teaspoon
A hand palm	=	3 ounces
A fist	=	1 cup
A handful	=	1 to 2 ounces of snack food

—K. McNutt, *Nutrition Today* 28(5) (1993): 41–43.

Up the Servings for High-Energy Need

Individuals with high-caloric needs must increase the number of servings. An extremely active male with a caloric requirement twice as high as in the above diet needs to get extra food. Such a diet would include more servings from the grain group and include more vegetables and fruits as well as a number of items from the empty calorie group. In the United States, most adults require anywhere between 1,600 and 2,800 Calories, depending on the body size and activity. In general a small inactive person would be on the lower end of the energy requirement while a large extremely active person would land on the high end of energy requirement. The numbers of servings from each food group for three different energy levels are given in table 5. Note that the number of servings from the dairy group stay the same across caloric levels, meats increase some, while the grains have almost doubled. The reason of course is the grain group is the major calorie source in our diets. Rapidly growing children, especially those during the adolescent growth spurt, need more calories and nutrients, and a rapidly growing physically active teenage boy may need even more than 2,800 Calories. The person's appetite should be the guide as long as wholesome foods from the food groups are selected.

Table 5

More Servings with Increasing Caloric Needs

Calories Per Day	Veges	Fruits	Grains	Dairy*	Meat
1,600	3	2	6	2	5
2,200	4	3	9	2	6
2,800	5	4	11	2	7

*Women who are pregnant or breastfeeding, teenagers, and young adults to age twenty-four need three servings.

—S. Welch et al., *Nutrition Today* 27(6) (1992): 12–23.

A *calorie* is a unit expressing heat or energy value of food. Calories come from carbohydrate, protein, fat, and alcohol.

One great advantage of eating according to the food guide is the flexibility to modify the diet in terms of calories and nutrients. For example, an excellent weight-reduction program would be to increase one's exercise and to select the low-calorie diet (1,600 Cal, table 5) with the least dietary fat. By decreasing the fat you can lower the calories even further to bring down your diet to as low as 1,200 Cal. Such diets will provide nutrients and at the same time limit calories. Eating three meals with some protein foods at every meal will almost always prevent ravenous food-seeking behavior, which often plays havoc with weight-reduction diets.

Step Three: Go Forward with Your Own Diet Plan

Now that you know how to evaluate your food intake and have a baseline of your daily food, you need to start planning your own diet. The first point is to select the recommended servings from each of the food groups. Second, you need to select the serving sizes suggested for each food. Keep foods from the fat/sugar/alcohol group low, at least initially.

The number of servings you must choose from each food group depends on your energy requirement. Your physical activity and body size will determine how much you need. A physically active person needs more energy than a sedentary person, and a tall person has a greater energy need than a small-sized individual.

In table 6, diets based on the food guide are given at three caloric levels. If you are a small inactive person, 1,600 Calories or less would be adequate for you. A physically active person of average height would need in the order of 2,200 Calories and a young teenager, still growing and extremely active, would require as much as 2,800 Calories or more.

Table 6

Diet Sampler Based on the Food Guide
for Three Calorie Levels

Calories Per Day	1,600	2,200	2,800
Breakfast	2 grain	3 grain	4 grain
	1 fruit	1 fruit	2 fruit
	1 dairy	1 dairy	1 dairy
Lunch	2 grain	3 grain	3 grain
	1 veges	2 veges	3 veges
	3 meat	4 meat	4 meat
	1 fruit	1 fruit	1 fruit
Supper	2 grain	3 grain	4 grain
	2 veges	2 veges	2 veges
	2 meat	2 meat	3 meat
		1 fruit	1 fruit
Snack	1 dairy	1 dairy	1 dairy
			1 fruit
Total fat in grams	53	73	93

Let's now assume you are a small, inactive person. The lowest calorie level of the food guide sample in table 6 would be the most appropriate. A diet of six grain, two fruit, three vegetable, two dairy, and five meat servings is recommended. You can distribute these servings any way you like during the day, but a regular meal pattern as is suggested in table 6 is better for you.

With increasing activity and body size, your caloric need also increases. Note through that the servings from the dairy group do not increase since two servings are recommended over the whole range of energy intake. While fruit, vegetable, and meat servings only slightly increase, the bread/grain/cereal group increases dramatically to as many as eleven servings for the 2,800-Cal diet. This makes sense since the major portion of our calories should come from the grain group.

After you have selected the diet that most approximates your situation, select the foods with their appropriate serving sizes you want to include in your daily menu. For most items serving sizes are easily recognizable portions. A slice of bread, six ounces of orange juice, an apple, a cup of milk are portions used by many of us on a regular basis. *New are the small serving sizes for the meat group.* To call one egg, or half a cup of baked beans a serving is understandable. But we need to relearn that ONE OUNCE of beef, pork, lamb, chicken or fish is equivalent to ONE SERVING. Three ounces of lean hamburger patty, half a cup of baked beans, and one egg would be your day's allotment from the meat group on the lowest calorie diet, for example. Furthermore the recommendations call for lean meat. Consequently, all meat must be well trimmed and have little marbling. You would remove the skin from chicken and turkey and cook your meat with no or little fat. The reason for this stringent use of lean meats is to keep the saturated fats to a minimum, yet obtain the protein, iron, vitamin B_{12}, and other nutrients present in these high-protein foods.

Other significant sources of saturated fats are dairy products, foremost butter, whole milk, cheeses, and all kinds of other dairy products, such as ice creams. Label reading will give you the fat content of milk, yogurt, cottage and riccota cheese, and the selection of low-fat dairy products is not difficult. A problem is the extraordinary number of cheeses on the market for which the fat content is not always given. In general, hard cheeses have lowered fat content.

With these ideas in mind, you can now plan your own diet. If you prepare food just for yourself, follow the number of servings and keep the fat as low as possible. If you prepare meals for several people, you need to take into account different energy needs. Let's assume a wife needs a 1,500-Cal diet while her husband needs 2,200 and her teenage son 2,800 Cal per day. If all three ate the same diet, the wife would end up obese, the husband might be all right, but the son would probably be underweight. To handle such a situation, the servings must be adjusted. By sticking to the servings of the 1,600-Cal diet and limiting the fat in her diet, the wife would obtain a low-calorie diet with adequate nutrients. The husband could eat the extra servings in between meals as snacks or help himself to extra servings from the bread, vegetable, fruit, and meat group. The teenager's diet would include even more of these helpings, which can be served at mealtime or as snacks.

Specifics for You to Do

1. Select the daily calorie level that most approximates your situation.
2. Make up a day's menu for you based on the Food Guide.
3. If you prepare food for several people who have differing energy needs, make a food plan to compensate for these.

Optional: Evaluation of Our Sample Diet

After you have put together your own diet, go back to the "one day diet sample" given in this chapter to see whether eating from the food groups provides us with a healthful diet. The nutrient analysis given in table 7 was done using a simple computer program. It shows some very interesting points:

First question: *What are the calories in this diet and how can they be changed if we need more or less?*

Our computer printout tells us that this diet provides us with approximately 1,600 Cal per day. Such a diet would be about right for a female, sixty-six years of age, who weighs 62 kg (136 lbs), is five foot, four inches tall and lives a sedentary lifestyle. However, most individuals need more calories. Men and women leading active lives, or teenagers who are still growing, need many more calories. For higher calorie needs, all that is required is to increase

47

the servings mainly from the grain group. Get more servings of fruits and vegetables and slightly more servings from the meat group. On the other hand, if you need to reduce your calories below 1,600 per day, cut the fat and other items from the empty calorie group, making sure you receive the servings from the five food groups. This would give you a very low-calorie diet with a good balance of nutrients.

Table 7

Sample Diet Given in This Chapter
(Food/One Day)

0.5 cup	Corn flakes cereal—Kellogg's
0.5 cup	1% low-fat milk
6 oz	Orange juice, fresh
1 cup	Brewed coffee
3 oz	Chicken breast, meat-rstd.
0.5 cup	Iceberg lettuce, chopped
2 pce	Whole-wheat bread, 35 g
0.5 ea	Banana
2 cup	Tea from instant, unswtnd.
1 cup	White rice, regular/cooked
0.5 cup	Broccoli, chp, ckd f/raw
0.5 cup	Carrots, bld, drnd, w/o salt
0.5 cup	Red, kidney beans, ckd f/dry
1 ea	Whole egg, fried in marg.
1 ea	Apple w/peel, 2.75 in diam.
1 cup	Low-fat plain yogurt, 12 g
4 ea	Whole-grain rye crackers
1 oz	Swiss cheese
1 tsp	Low-cal French dressing
1 tsp	Olive oil
2 tsp	Butter, unsalted

(continued on next page)

Table 7 (continued)

Nutrients in Sample Diet	Amounts	RDA
Calories	1612	1623
Protein	87.5 G	53.1 G
Carbohydrates	233 G	235 G
Dietary fiber	27.8 G	16.2 G
Fat Total	40 G	54 G
Saturated	17.3 G	18 G
Mono	14.3 G	18 G
Poly	5.07 G	18 G
Cholesterol	351 mg	300 mg*
A-carotene	2091 RE	
A-preformed	507 RE	
A-Total	2599 RE	800 RE
Thiamin, B_1	1.42 mg	1 mg
Riboflavin, B_2	1.881 mg	1.2 mg
Niacin, B_3	22.6 mg	13 mg
Vitamin B_6	2.24 mg	1.6 mg
Vitamin B_{12}	2.92 mcg	2 mcg
Folacin	409 mcg	180 mcg
Pantothenic	6.04 mg	7 mg
Vitamin C	169 mg	60 mg
Vitamin E	6.65 mg	8 mg
Calcium	1120 mg	800 mg
Copper	1.17 mg	2.5 mg
Iron	13.0 mg	10 mg
Magnesium	356 mg	280 mg

*Limited to less than 300mg/day.

(continued on next page)

Table 7 (continued)

Phosphorus	1528 mg	800 mg
Potassium	3239 mg	2000 mg
Selenium	115 mcg	55 mcg
Sodium	1394 mg	2400 mg
Zinc	12.3 mg	12 mg

Calories from protein:	21%
Calories from carbohydrates:	57%
Calories from fats:	22%
Calories from other:	0%

Second question: *Is the nutrient content of our one-day diet sample adequate?*

The nutrient amounts on our computer printout compare favorably with the nutrient RDAs. Just run down the figures and compare them with the RDAs for protein, vitamins, and minerals. Our diet provides more than enough protein, three times the amount of vitamin A and vitamin C, while all other vitamins and minerals are present in acceptable concentrations.

Our third question: *Is the diet a healthful one?*

The total amount of fats you use daily and the type of fat you select is the 64 thousand dollar question. As we have seen in prior sections, the major health issues relate to the amount and type of fat, to fiber, cholesterol, salt and alcohol in the diet. Let's take one at a time.

The total *fat intake* is quite low, forty grams of fat per day. This is quite low, and for most people, this could be increased. But we need to remember that even a small amount of fat will increase the calories by a ratio of nine (one gram fat provides nine calories). Fat intake, as all other nutrients, will vary from day to day. If the next day we choose a hamburger steak instead of chicken, we automatically get more fat. Such day-to-day variations are to be expected.

Sometimes the calories from fat are expressed as a percentage of total calories. In our sample the fat calories make up 22 percent. This is a very low value and much lower than usual American intakes, which have been as high as 45 percent. Many people have had difficulties doing something about these high fat intakes. In our sample, planned according to the Food Guide, fat almost automatically is low. Starting with a diet without foods from the empty calorie category, we have leeway and actually can increase the fat over and above the basic diet.

Another point about fat is the *importance of the type of fat.* If you check the breakdown into saturated, monos, and polyunsaturated fats, you see that they are represented in different amounts. In diets where the fat comes predominantly from dairy and meats, we have a preponderance of saturated fats. In our example the saturated fat comes from butter, milk, cheese, and chicken. On this particular day, the saturated fat outweighs the monos and polys. We get polys from oils and deep-sea fish. If on the following day we include a piece of salmon or other deep sea fish instead of chicken or beef and substitute margarine for butter, the fat composition of our diet would be more in favor of the polys.

Many American diets are quite *low in fiber,* and values of five to eight grams per day are common. Compared to such values, our basic diet sample is a good source of dietary fiber with almost 28 grams. In our sample the fiber comes from kidney beans, whole grain bread, vegetables, and fruits.

If you check the *dietary cholesterol* intake, you will find a value of 351 mg per day. Cholesterol is not a nutrient and because it can contribute to increased blood cholesterol levels, we want to keep the dietary cholesterol on the low side. The American Heart Association recommends an upper level of approximately 300 mg per day. With our sample diet, we are somewhat above the cut-off level because we have included an egg as part of our daily menu. As long as we limit the eggs to two per week, this one day excess will even out.

The sodium in our sample is low. This reflects that no processed foods and extra salt had been added to our diet. Bread, crackers, salad dressing, butter, cheese, and milk are foods that all contribute some salt. To flavor vegetables and meats, spices and herbs and some salt can be used. The inclusion of processed meats, pickles, cold cuts, canned vegetables, on the other hand, would increase the sodium content considerably. Our body conserves sodium very efficiently, but some sodium in our diet is necessary. Since many of the foods we consume contain some natural salt, the salt shaker on the table is usually not necessary. Too much salt in a food actually hides the natural flavor of the food.

Our diet sample does not contain any *alcoholic beverages*. If any is included, moderation is key. Check the calories from alcohol. They are empty calories. Some connoisseurs claim that beer and certain wines provide us with some nutrients. For practical purpose and intent, this is stretching the point. It is more appropriate to obtain nutrients from food. Furthermore, strong alcoholic drinks consumed on an empty stomach can damage the gastrointestinal lining, resulting in reduced absorption of nutrients from other food.

Using the food guide with a minimum of planning allows us to put together varied and healthful diets that provide a remarkable balance of the essential nutrients and calories according to individual needs. Furthermore, by limiting food items from the fat/sugar/salt/alcohol group, we create healthful diets, which are beneficial in decreasing the risk of chronic disease.

For Contrast Just Consider This

If you find eating from the food group boring or too much work, consider the following daily food intake. It is a diet consumed not too uncommonly. In three meals the following foods were eaten:

Breakfast: 2 cups of coffee with cream and sugar
    1 doughnut, jelly filled

Lunch: 1 cheeseburger
    4 oz chocolate milkshake
Supper: 1 pork chop
    1 baked potato with skin
    2 dill pickles
    half a fresh tomato
    2 cups coffee with cream
    1 piece of apple pie

This diet provided: 3,730 Cal, 271 g fat, 11 g dietary fiber, 829 mg cholesterol. It is not known how long it takes on such fare to become obese and develop atheroslerosis.

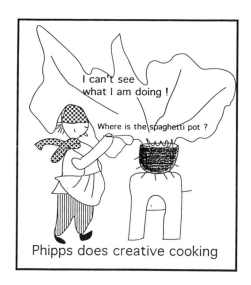

Phipps does creative cooking

Chapter V
Creative Cooking

Hardly any day goes by without exposure by the media to mouth-watering foods or meals. Many of the lucullan meals shown in newspapers and ads are in actual fact pictures of plastic models, but they show that food attractively presented appeals to our senses. If you prepare a meal, you need to consider the appeal it has for the person who will eat it, in addition to its nutritional quality and its cost. In general, home cooking with basic ingredients is the most economic and we know exactly what ingredients are used. Let's assume you are taking care of your own or your family's meals. How do you go about preparing them?

Table 8

Where Americans Get Their Nutrition Information

17,000 American women, aged sixteen–thirty-four, said they get their nutrition information from:*

Magazines	86%
Food packages	53%
Books	52%
Friends and family	34%
Other media	26%
Physician	15%
Exercise instructor	11%
Government publications	8%
Other nutritionist	8%
Registered dietitian	7%

—J. Kirby, *Nutrition Today* 29(3) (1994): 6–9.

*Numbers add up to more than 100 percent because of multiple responses.

A Nutritious Food-Buying Spree

To make nutritious, flavorful meals that are appealing, you need to start with quality food. To prevent impulse buying, prepare a shopping list with the items you need to buy. Even if you have an excellent memory and will remember what you need, a shopping list is helpful. You may not always buy exactly what's on your list. Flexibility is necessary to take advantage of special bargains and seasonal items when they appear on the market. The shopping list is also a reminder to buy all you need and to prevent multiple trips to the market for items you forgot to buy.

Many items are bought on a regular basis, such as milk or bread, so it is advantageous to develop a basic list, which can be used routinely. Imagine the layout of your supermarket and organize the items you need and want to buy accordingly, for example, fruits and vegetables near the entrance of the market, meats and deli items next, then cereals and breads, etc. As you go along your shopping route, compare prices for economic advantage and learn to use the nutrition information on packaged foods.

To assure your buying foods for varied, balanced, and moderate diets, the shopping list will have to show predominately items from the five food groups, with a considered and possibly limited selection of items from the empty calorie group.

Items that are a must on your shopping list:
Vegetables. Buy yellow and green vegetables. Veges should look fresh, not wilted. Canned vegetables may be high in salt.
Fruits and Fruit Juices. Select a good vitamin C source. Buy fruits in season. Do not substitute drinks for the real juice. Canned fruits can be high in sugar.
Grain / Cereals / Bread. Select some of the whole grain types as a good source of fiber. Check cereals for sugar content; use sweets, cookies, rich cakes sparingly or only on special occasions.
Meats, Chicken, Turkey, and Fish. Select low-fat cuts for freshness, tuna packed in water. Go slow on high fat,

high salt items, such as hot dogs, bacon, and ham and most cold cuts.

Legumes. Select low-cost protein from baked beans, lentils, split peas.

Eggs. Adults use about two per week/person.

Milk/Dairy. Select fat-controlled products, appropriate for your need.

Fats, oils. Use butter and margarine very sparingly. Use olive oil or another oil for cooking. Any oil on the market can be used as salad dressing.

Sugar. Use sparingly, as sweetener only. Beware of rich sugary foods.

Add other items to your shopping list, as required, such as beverages, canned goods, cleaning articles, etc. Go slow on cookies, candies, and highly processed foods.

Estimates show that each one of us spends significant amounts of money on food. Almost everybody, except perhaps a few, must live on fixed budgets and needs to spend food dollars carefully. Unit pricing helps compare prices of foods of different brands and quantities. So does buying what is advertised during special sales. Fruits and vegetables in season are sometimes cheaper. Although special offers can save money, if you don't use the item properly, it may not be a good buy. If you are hungry when you go shopping, you probably buy more than you actually need. Hunger overrides your good judgment, especially when food looks enticing.

Your income will determine how much you spend on food. With limiting finances it is vital to know how to get the most nutritious food from your food dollar. To prepare frugal and delicious meals, use basic foods. Cooked oatmeal for breakfast is cheaper than packaged cereals. In general, foods prepared from scratch are cheaper and often more nutritious than processed foods. On the other hand, many prepared foods, for example, baked beans, tomato soup, canned juice-packed pineapple, can be very useful additions to your menus. The frugal shopper needs to compare food prices, evaluate food quality, and read nutrition labels. Food advertisements can be helpful but need to be evaluated on their merit.

The New Food Label as a Tool for Healthy Eating

The percent daily value (DV) shows how a food fits into the overall daily diet. Higher percentages mean greater amounts of nutrients. For most people the goal is to choose foods that add up to 100 percent DV or more for total carbohydrate, dietary fiber, and the vitamins and minerals, and 100 percent or less for total fat, saturated fat, cholesterol, and sodium.
—E. Saltos, et al. *Nutrition Today* 29 (1994): 19–22.

Microbes Can Kill

When you get home from the market, store the food immediately to retain the nutritional quality and to prevent food decay. Grain products when dry can be stored for longer periods while breads—especially the whole grain ones—can get moldy. Refrigeration retards spoilage. Highly perishable vegetables and fruits are best stored in the refrigerator, while root vegetables and potatoes are kept in a cool, dry, dark place, care being taken to open cellophane wrappers to let the vegtables come in contact with air. The proper care of vegetables and fruits is usually learned quickly by trial and error. Fresh produce is more appetizing and has superior nutritional value.

Proper Food Handling Is Important

In the United States, 9,000 deaths each year are linked to eating contaminated food. Estimated cost to U.S. economy $5 billion.
—M. Doyle, *Nutrition Reviews* 51 (1993): 346–347.

Dairy products need to be refrigerated. Meats and chicken spoil quickly; they can be frozen if you buy them in bulk. Separate in portions before freezing so that you can defrost only as much as you need for a meal. Leftovers from a meal need to be refrigerated promptly. Sometimes leftovers are planned to be used at a second meal or in soups (leftover noodles in tomato soup, pieces of chicken on toast, etc.). With modern conveniences, storage of food is no problem and much time can be saved by shopping only once or twice per week. Experience over a period of time will help you decide what works best for you. Everybody has different food likes, ideas, and circumstances and you need to take these into account.

Foods that are moist and full of nutrients, such as a vegeatble stew, must be refrigerated promptly because they spoil easily. Such foods are also "good food" for a host of bacteria and microorganisms, such as salmonella, botulinus, molds, and other microbes that attack food and can harm us when we eat such contaminated food. The ambient temperature range in which we feel most comfortable is also the optimum temperature for microbes to grow most rapidly, and therefore food is most susceptible to microbial spoilage at room temperature. When food smells sour or has an off flavor, it should be discarded. A special problem is the growth of *C. botulinum,* which does not advertise its presence by an objectionable smell. This microbe grows under air exclusion as in canned, bottled, or tightly covered foods. Microbially spoilt foods will give you a headache and diarrhea within a day or so. Similar symptoms are experienced in botulism, which is further complicated by the production of toxins that can kill (see figure 3).

Plan First-Class Meals

To establish regular meal patterns, it is helpful to make sure each person will obtain the necessary food and that eating is not left to a haphazard eating routine. Depending on the type of food, a meal takes between three and five hours to be digested after which hunger feelings return. Hunger occurs when the stomach is empty and contracts, sometimes leading to painful hunger pangs. Well-spaced meals, especially for children and teenagers,

TEMPERATURE OF FOOD
for control of food poisoning bacteria

°F		
212		BOILING
	Kills most bacteria	COOKING
165		
	Prevents most bacterial growth	WARMING
140		
125	Allows some bacterial growth	
	Rapid bacterial growth Toxins produced	DANGER
60		
	Allows some bacterial growth	THAWING
40		
32	Slows bacterial growth	REFRIGERATING
	Stops bacterial growth	FREEZING
0		

Figure 3

prevent excessive hunger episodes. Hunger is a powerful stimulus and may lead to ravenous appetites and food-seeking behavior. After a meal one feels satiated. When the food is digested, hunger slowly returns. Well-spaced meals give the right balance between hunger and satiation without either becoming excessive.

The conventional meal pattern in the United States has consisted of three meals: breakfast, lunch, and dinner/supper with in-between snacks for children and beverages for adults. A new two-meal pattern has evolved for some individuals who rise late in the morning and combine breakfast and lunch. There are a good number of people who just eat when they think about it, or have no specific time and place for their meals. Whatever patterns a person chooses, the food eaten is always part of the whole day's diet. If you skip breakfast, you most likely miss out on the traditional orange juice. A snack during the day could make up for this. In theory it is possible to get all nutrients from snacks, but usually snack foods are high in calories, salt, sugar, and are often refined foods. Whether you eat regular meals or whether you predominantly snack, the day's food intake must meet a person's nutritional needs.

To encourage the flow of digestive juices, attention must be given to the sensory qualities of food. The smell, the look, the taste, and flavor and consistency of food all play a part. Do you think a meal of white cauliflower, white rice, and boiled chicken breast looks appetizing? Would you not rather prefer broccoli, chicken in tomato sauce, and white rice for better eye appeal? By contrast our taste buds are overwhelmed with too many strong flavors, especially when they all are unique. Therefore, serve strong tasting foods with bland ones. Serve some foods hot, others cold. Too much of one or the other per meal is boring. Even in summer, when cold foods are preferred, a meal including one hot item adds interest. Food consistency is another point to keep in mind. A meal is made interesting if one food is crunchy, another mushy, and yet another soft. Variety in looks, flavor, texture, and even spatial arrangement of food on the plate are as important as the nutritional value of food.

The setting a meal is served in also affects our well being. Even highly frugal meals can be eaten in congenial settings. Since cooking a meal requires attention, it is helpful to lay the table before starting to cook. Use colorful tableware, spotless dishes and cutlery, and make sure all eating utensils are at hand. It is unpleasant to have to get up several times during the meal.

When you prepare a meal, expect that different people have individual taste preferences. Highly nutritious foods with unfamiliar tastes will in most cases be wasted. Taste preferences are formed early in life, and the introduction to different flavors, tastes, and textures should occur during childhood. The appetizing serving of foods may tempt a person to try an unfamiliar food, but in most cases once food habits are established, relearning takes time.

Cooking Advice Tailormade to Your Need

The opportunitites to learn to cook and prepare meals are endless. Gourmet demonstration on TV, in evening classes, cooking recipes in women's magazines abound, as well as recipes on food packages. In addition markets are now specializing in selling whole dinners. Salad bars offer a large variety of salads and raw vegetables. The bakery section sells a variety of breads, bagels, crumpets and muffins. Opportunities for the ease of obtaining meals without even trying one's hand at cooking or baking are endless.

However, preparing food on one's own is a very satisfying experience and many individuals and families cannot afford the greater expense of ready-made foods. Some want to avoid excessive additives, others want to know what goes into food, and others again like the taste of home-cooked food. When starting to try one's hand at cooking, it is helpful to begin with several basic, comparatively easy recipes, which allow modification. Knowledge of cooking techniques for vegetables is important because they are often overcooked. Stir-frying of vegetables has come into vogue. Cooking time is short and nutrients are retained, but often too much oil and fat are added. A large frypan will do if you do not have a wok. Nutrients are retained best if vegetables are briefly steamed with little water. Use a watch to time the cooking period for best results. When vegetables are done to perfection, flavor with a little (not too much) oil, which adds extra flavor and aids in the absorption of fat-soluble vitamins and beta-carotene from the vegetables. (In stir-frying, you'd begin with a small amount of oil in the frying pan or wok so you wouldn't need to add any more oil.)

A few of the many tasteful vegetable combinations are: green, red, and yellow pepper cut in strips, steamed a few minutes, seasoned with little oil; similarly prepared are:

zucchini, yellow summer squash, and tomato;
green pepper, onion, and tomato;
shredded cabbage, grated carrots, and minced green pepper.

All kinds of herbs, fresh or dried, give added flavor. Experiment with herbs and spices to find the flavors you like best. Vegetables are naturally low in salt. Too much added salt smothers the natural taste of the freshly cooked vegetables (see table 9).

Table 9

Herbs Give Flavor to Foods

Sweet or dried basil	Used with tomato, chicken, fish, vegetables, salads
Bay leaves (Laurel)	In stews, with meats, fish, poultry, vegetables
Oregano	Tomato dishes, pizza, meats, soups, egg
Rosemary	Stews, soups, vegetables
Sage	Poultry seasoning, fish, salads
Thyme	Fish, meats, poultry, vegetables, fresh tomato
Tarragon	Salad dressings, vegetables, meats, fish

The cooking of meats requires knowledge of broiling, steaming, baking, and many other ways of preparation. Unfortunately the best meat cuts contain in general the most fat (see table 1 for the six leanest meats). The tougher meat cuts are nutritionally more desirable because they are usually leaner. Such cuts can be boiled and used in stews. The ability to make a good stew is one of the basic skills, which comes in very handy. Cook the meat in water with some flavorful vegetables (onions, celery, carrots, parsley, and a bay leaf), let the stew cool, and skim off the fat. Then add barley or rice and lastly add the vegetables you want to add. Especially in winter, stews are a good way of preparing meat with a low fat content together with grains, potato, and all the vegetables desired.

Knowing how to cook chicken and fowl is another basic skill. Roasted, broiled, braised, and boiled methods offer a large variety of different dishes that provide a good protein source. If you have once roasted a chicken, you will be impressed by how easy it is and leftovers can be used in sandwiches, salads, or may be frozen and used at a later date. While cooking fish is not difficult, it is important that this food be fresh. Fish that has an off smell and an unappetizing look may be a health hazard and can give you food poisoning. Buy fish from a good fish store and use canned tuna once opened and other canned seafood immediately. Tuna packed in water with a little added mayonnaise, chopped celery and shredded lettuce, is a food liked by young and old.

The Confusing World of Cookbooks

The number and type of cookbooks on the market are truly staggering, and it may be difficult to select the one that will best serve your need. Cookbooks have been classified into major groupings by Todhunter (1992). Kitchen books give useful information on how to prepare every type of food. Armchair books are cookbooks that are enjoyable to read and give information also on the history of foods throughout the ages. Other types are bedside books, coffee-table books, and those that have collectors' value.

The cookbooks sold widely are those that are written and advertised by television personalities.

Today the sale of cookbooks is exceeded only by sales of the Bible and dictionaries.
    —E.N. Todhunter, *Nutrition Today* 27 (1) (1992): 6–12.

"Cookbooks sell because food is a common denominator of interest to everyone," according to Todhunter. Many newer versions of cookbooks, the one published by Oprah, for example, give some nutrition information, such as the calories and fat in a food. As fascinating and useful as cookbooks are, when you follow their recipes, you need to keep your total diet in mind. If one of your favorite recipes temporarily is wrecking your healthful eating pattern, it may be of minor concern. However, a diet that is made up of a series of very high fat gourmet recipes will eventually take its toll. If you like a food that calls for ingredients heavily drawn from the high sugar, high fat group, and requires much added salt, use your imagination and modify the recipe, using more acceptable ingredients.

To Drink or Not to Drink Is the Question

Unsweetened beverages as coffee, tea, seltzer water do not provide nutrients but are an important source of fluid. Water is so plentiful and our thirst mechanism works so well that usually we take it for granted. Beverages and juices that are also nutrient sources, such as orange or tomato juice, must be counted as part of your daily diet. This also is true for high sugar or alcoholic drinks which provide only empty calories and no nutrients. Such drinks increase the portions you receive from the sixth food group (see table 10).

Table 10

Sugar Content of Common Beverages

		Sugar (g)	Approx oz	Number of Teaspoons
Pepsi-Cola	8 oz	27.6	1	6
Coca-Cola	1 bottle	20.4	2/3	4–5
Ginger ale	8 oz	20.7	2/3	4–5
Carbonated	1 bottle	20.4	2/3	4–5
From Food Composition Table				

Individuals who have small appetites should drink water or a beverage between meals. Their appetite may decrease rapidly when they ingest fluid at the start of a meal. Most people like a beverage with a meal, either hot or cold, depending on the season or preference. Water is one of the best thirst-quenching drinks, and children should get used to its taste and drink enough, especially during the hot season.

Food on the Table, Bon Appetit, and Relax

To bring a meal on the table requires the coordination of many activities. When you prepare a meal, start with the food item that takes longest to cook. Defrost frozen items in the refrigerator ahead of time. When you start cooking, put the kettle on immediately in order to have hot water ready for steaming vegetables or rice, etc. Prepare everything before you start—such as cutting vegetables, trimming meat, getting salad greens washed. Lay the table before you start to cook and get dishes warmed up and the cutlery ready. If you bake a chicken, use the oven to roast potatoes, or to bake a dessert at the same time. Organization is essential, especially if you have limited time. A good meal for four, if organized well, can be made in thirty minutes (if the chicken was put in the oven an hour or so before). As you cook your meal, make it a habit to clean your cooking utensils immediately after you have used them. Wipe your countertop clean when you have finished a job. Pots and pans with dried-on food are harder to scrub clean than a pot that has been soaked in water and soap. There is no need for the kitchen to look like a battlefield after every meal. Tasting foods during cooking is necessary for some dishes. Have a tasting spoon, which is rinsed after each tasting. It is unappetizing and not hygienic when the cook samples food without washing the spoon.

A meal should be eaten with leisure. Don't air your daily problems during a meal. Food should be appreciated, and the atmosphere should be friendly. Children need to be encouraged, but not forced, to eat a varity of foods. In addition, table manners need to be learned. Eating a variety of foods, eating moderately, acquiring table manners, all are learning processes, which are strongly modeled by parents.

Step Four: Meals from Scratch

Today we are interested in food shopping and preparation. You may prepare all or part of your meals or you may eat out. In any case selecting nourishing food is a must. In terms of food planning, it makes a difference whether you live alone or in a group. Official data show that a single person spends considerably more money on food than a person as a member of a group or family. In part this is due to bulk buying. Food planning is often influenced by the availability of food. If a market is nearby, you might want to go shopping more frequently than you would if you live miles from the nearest supermarket. Also make sure you have some nonperishable foods in stock for unforeseen occasions. A friend may drop by unexpectedly, or you cannot get to the market because of a hurricane or snowstorm.

Just once in your life, take the time to go through each step outlined above. Food shopping and preparation is an art, and everybody should know how to put a simple meal together. There are very few of us who have the luxury of having all our meals prepared. If food shopping and preparation is something you do all the time and have much experience, skip this section. Once you have done it several times, it will become second nature to you and much of what you do becomes automatic. After you have checked what food you still have at home, decide what you need to buy and prepare your shopping list. Start with the number of servings you need for each food group per person per week. This will give you a rough estimate how much to buy. Let's assume you need two servings of fruit per day and shop for a week for just one person. You would have to buy a total of fourteen servings per week for example: seven oranges (1 per day), two bananas (1/2 per day), two apples, and one pear. The same considerations apply for the other food groups. The first time around, it will take a little time to work out some of the amounts you need.

Shopping for food requires alertness. At the supermarket, constantly evaluate foods for price, freshness, and quality. When expensive items are bought, identify whether you get convenient portions out of it. Estimate possible leftovers and what to do with them. Be flexible. Pay special attention to perishable items. Only buy as much as you can use immediately. If you have the choice of several markets, find out what their specialties are. One may have especially fine bread, another extra fresh vegetables.

When you have shopped and stored your food properly, you are ready for food preparation. Keep portions in mind. Cooking is a challenge, it sometimes can be great fun, but often it is a job that needs perseverance. During these times we need to remember that our food is health-giving and is important for our well-being. In the long run, it is cheaper than the medical costs of chronic disease.

Mastering the planning, cooking, and serving of food takes time. Gaining experience is a slow process of trial and error. Occasionally we get tired of the constant push to come up with three meals per day. For times when meal preparation becomes a drag, have some simple recipes ready that will save time and effort and yet are liked, or else celebrate and eat out as a treat.

A final thought on meal planning. Companies specializing in food for institutions, such as hospitals, colleges, the army, and large restaurants often use what is called cycle menus. Cycle menus may run three weeks, during which time well worked-out meals are prepared without repeating foods, except of course the staples like bread or milk. After three weeks the cycle begins anew and this way of excellent planning variety is achieved with high efficiency. Different cycle menus are worked out for different seasons to use seasonal foods.

While cycle menus are too inflexible for small units, such as a family or a single person, the idea of writing down a set of menus for the week is a good idea. Collect a series of basic food recipes that have worked well in the past for you. Modify some of the basic recipes in accord with good nutrition and taste preference. This is also a convenient way to use leftovers. Take, for example, a stew. You can make a delicious meal with all kinds of vegetables "thrown in." You also need some recipes for quick meals you can whip up in practically no time at all in an emergency or at a time when your strength is at a low ebb.

For You to Do as Part of *Step Four* Exercise

1. How much money did you spend on your food per week?
2. What is the average time you take to prepare a meal?
3. Was all the food you bought used to good advantage or did you have to throw away any food?
4. Was your food selection in accord with eating the recommended servings from the food groups?
5. Did you have a problem with any of the steps outlined above?

   · Do you need better cooking skills?
   · Is your kitchen equipment in good shape?
   · Do you need to improve cleanliness and hygiene when you prepare food?
   · Is your refrigerator in good working order, clean and organized?

Make a list of the improvements you feel you should make, and set yourself a time frame in which to accomplish them.

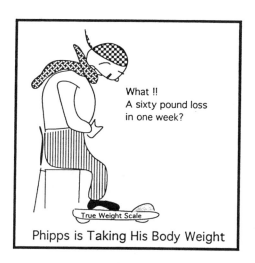

What !!
A sixty pound loss
in one week?

True Weight Scale

Phipps is Taking His Body Weight

Chapter VI
Checkpoint Body Weight

An important tool in evaluating a person's overall nutrition is body weight. In a child repeated weight and height measurements will show whether the diet is adequate for optimum growth. In adults, body weight indicates whether a person is over- or under-weight, but more importantly serial weighing over a period of time will show whether a person's weight is stable and energy intake matches energy output. Loss of weight indicates insufficient dietary calories to cover energy needs. Body weight increases signal creeping obesity due to more calories taken in by diet than are used for body needs and activity.

One seemingly all-pervasive concern today is the desire for the "ideal" body weight. Adults and even children are concerned about it. Unfortunately body weight is one of the most misunder-stood concepts. Preoccupation with it has resulted in misdirected lifestyles, senseless dieting, money wasted on useless diet aids, heartache and unhappiness when diets did not work. In some societies the accepted body weight norms are very different from those in the U.S., and the "ideal body weight" is very much dependent on societal factors. The super-thin, willowy slender body image fashion models portray in advertisements and the media is unrealistic and misleading for the general population. Yet many women aspire to it, although there is no proof that such individuals are healthier.

In any population heights and body weights of individuals of the same age and gender vary. This is quite natural. Everybody is unique in terms of height and weight. Science tells us that people vary in their muscle size and also in their fat tissue. By exercising and good nutrition, we can increase our muscle mass to a small degree while in caloric overnutrition, our fat tissue becomes excessive resulting in obesity. Good energy stores, such as fat under our skin and around internal organs, have been beneficial during times of food shortages in the past. In modern affluent societies, excessive storage of fat serves no purpose and even is a health hazard.

ESCAPE THE FRUSTRATING WEIGHT-CYCLING TRAP

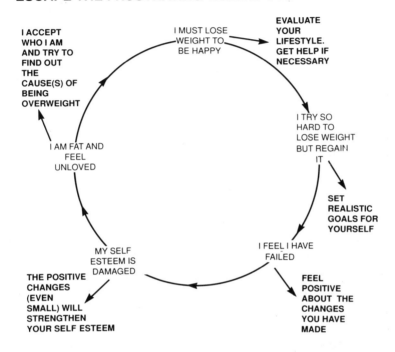

Figure 4

The Energy Balance Effect

Adults whose body weights are stable over long periods of time are in energy balance. The calories obtained from food are equal to the calories used for body processes and daily activities. Obesity is the result of too many calories obtained from food without using this energy in activity, such as walking, heavy work, playing games, or running. The causes of obesity are complex. Obesity has been related to genetic factors, hormonal imbalances, psychological or social factors, as well as habitual overeating and inactivity. Obesity taxes the heart and predisposes to hypertension, heart disease, stroke, diabetes, and gallstones among others. While we cannot alter our genetic makeup, we need to recognize the psychosocial factors that lead to obesity. Eating well-balanced diets, limiting empty calories, in particular too much fat, and exercising regularly can help towards preventing it.

Conversely too few calories consumed in relation to the calories expended will lead to loss of weight. Such a situation can occur if a person who is in energy balance suddenly decides to exercise more than usual or if the calories in the diet are reduced. Some people are naturally thin and appear underweight, but severe underweight is a health hazard also. We are meant to carry some energy reserves as fat in our body, and women have naturally more fat than men. We draw on the stored fat between meals, and during exercise. The energy makes us more buoyant and enthusiastic, where otherwise we would literally drag ourselves through the day.

Useful Comparisons

In the U.S. the standards for weight and height frequently used by the medical community are those obtained from Metropolitan Life Insurance data (see figure 5). These reference weights came from men and women aged twenty-five to fifty-nine with the lowest mortality rates. Under A, "Desirable Body Weight Ranges" are given for men and women. In a newer 1990 version

Compare Yourself with Body Weight Standards*

Comparison of Body Weight Standards Proposed in Dietary Guidelines for Americans: A, 1985; B, 1990*

A. Desirable Body Weight Ranges†			B. Suggested Weights for Adults		
Height without Shoes	Weight without Clothes		Height without Shoes	Weight in Pounds without Clothes	
	Men (pounds)	Women (pounds)		19 to 34 Years	35 Years and Over
4'10"		92–121			
4'11"		95–124			
5'0"		98–127	5'0"	97–128‡	108–138
5'1"	105–134	101–130	5'1"	101–132	111–143
5'2"	108–137	104–134	5'2"	104–137	115–148
5'3"	111–141	107–138	5'3"	107–141	119–152
5'4"	114–145	110–142	5'4"	111–146	122–157
5'5"	117–149	114–146	5'5"	114–150	126–162
5'6"	121–154	118–150	5'6"	118–155	130–167
5'7"	125–159	122–154	5'7"	121–160	134–172
5'8"	129–163	126–159	5'8"	125–164	138–178
5'9"	133–167	130–164	5'9"	129–169	142–183
5'10"	137–172	134–169	5'10"	132–174	146–188
5'11"	141–177		5'11"	136–179	151–194
6'0"	145–182		6'0"	140–184	155–199
6'1"	149–187		6'1"	144–189	159–205
6'2"	153–192		6'2"	148–195	164–210
6'3"	157–197		6'3"	152–200	168–216
			6'4"	156–205	173–222
			6'5"	160–211	177–228
			6'6"	164–216	182–234

* Source A: Adapted from the 1959 Metropolitan Desirable Weight Table. B: Derived from National Research Council, 1989.

† Note: For women 18 to 25 years, subtract one pound for each year under 25.

‡ The higher weights in the ranges generally apply to men, who tend to have more muscle and bone; the lower weights more often apply to women, who have less muscle and bone.

Figure 5

*T. Vanitallie and A.P. Simopoulos, "Summary of a National Obesity and Weight Control Symposium," *Nutrition Today* 28 (4) (1993): 33–35, reprinted by permission.

of "Suggested Weights for Adults," lower weight ranges for adults nineteen to thirty-four years are given than for adults thirty-five and older. Weighing yourself at regular intervals will tell you whether your body weight is stable, or whether you are gaining or losing weight.

From your body weight (in kg) and your height (in meters) your body mass index (BMI) is computed (BMI = body weight/height squared). In figure 6 the BMIs of nineteen to twenty-seven are given for various weight and heights. To use this chart, use your height and weight and find your BMI on the chart. If your BMI falls below nineteen, underweight is a concern (check it out with your physician). If your weight falls above the BMI of twenty-five, overweight must be considered. Epidemiological data suggested that the risks for heart disease, hypertension, and several other chronic diseases are lowest at or around a BMI of twenty-one. If over time your BMI is changing upwards, exercise more and reduce empty calories in your diet (see Appendix C).

Lifestyle Changes—Danger Points

Whenever we make changes in our life that alter our circumstances, our food and exercise habits are likely to be affected also. Examples are, young people leaving home for college gaining as much as fifteen pounds in a few months. Couples setting up a household may change their dietary habits. Women after a pregnancy may put on fat excessively. The elderly after losing a lifelong spouse may rapidly become underweight, frail, and prone to sickness. Even such seemingly insignificant changes as moving from one place to another affect our lifestyle and how we eat. When any of these changes occur, a conscious effort must be made to review one's daily food intake and to make readjustements if necessary.

In a new situation, it is helpful to observe for a week or so what you have eaten. Look at your meal pattern and access to food. You can go back to the beginning of these chapters and look at the type and size of servings your diet provides based on the food guide. In addition to reviewing your dietary practices, you

76

Find Your Body Mass Index

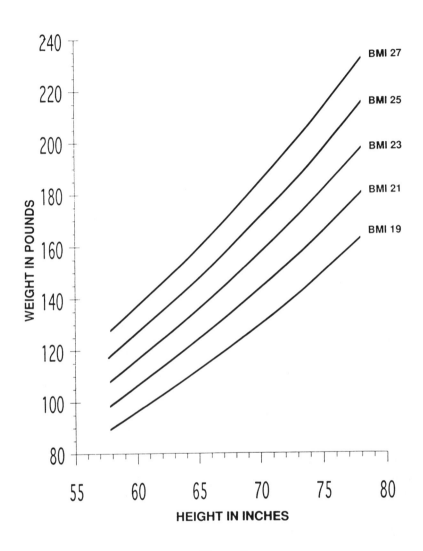

Figure 6

also need to check weekly body weights until you are confident that your diet, exercise, and general lifestyle are on track in the new setting. Such simple screening identifies problems with your diet, and you can prevent obesity before it gets out of hand.

Step Five: Your Weight Check

Your body weight should not become a fetish, but regular weighing is helpful in the identification of potential problems.

Adult body weights. Use a card or booklet to record your height and weight with the date. If you have a reasonably stable body weight, you can weigh yourself every two months, say on the first day of each other month. Weigh yourself on a good scale in the morning after emptying the bladder and with few clothes on and record the weight. If your weight is within two pounds of your last reading, you can assume you have been in energy balance.

If your weight has increased more than two pounds, watch it more closely at shorter intervals. If the increase is a true trend, start exercising and review your diet to adjust your dietary calories accordingly. Find out the reason for the change in your body weight. You may be rather inactive or your diet has changed, or you use food to console yourself during a difficult time. To prevent having to go on a weight-reduction program, act immediately. Prevention is better than treatment.

If you are not on a weight-reduction program and your body weight has decreased since your last weighing, also watch it closely. If the trend continues, you need to check out what the reason is for the weight loss. You may exercise too much, or you may not eat well, or you may be sick. Have the weight loss checked by your physician.

Adult body mass index. Find your BMI using your height and weight and read your value on the graph. If your BMI is in the twenty to twenty-five range, you do not need to make adjustments. If your BMI is approaching obesity (BMI above twenty-five, review your diet and activity and make adjustments by decreasing dietary calories and increasing physical activity. Individuals in the obese range need to evaluate their lifestyle and seek professional help to find out the cause(s) of the obesity. If you are underweight, have it checked by a physician.

Children's weight and height. Infants' and children's height/length and weight need to be taken periodically. When these measurements are plotted over a period of time on growth charts, they should fall either on one of the percentile levels or on a curve parallel to it. As long as height and weight fall on such lines, one can asssume that the child grows according to his/her unique growth pattern. Deviations from the usual parallel curve, either upward or downward, are of concern and need to be checked by the pediatrician. An upward trend in weight may signal beginning obesity; a downward trend may mean several things. The child may be sick, may not be getting enough food, may be too active, may be too tired to eat, or does not get the right foods (see Appendix D).

The first indications of obesity often occur during adolescence. Overweight adolescents should be screened for blood pressure, blood cholesterol, and concerns about weight, which, if necessary, should be followed by an in-depth medical assessment.

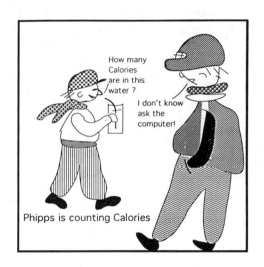

Chapter VII
The Energy in Foods

In earlier sections we have used the Food Guide to plan and prepare diets with variety, balance, and moderation. The result was a remarkably nutritious diet selected from a confusing number of foods. However, not all is well since the nutrients within each food group vary. Particular concern relates to the total calories and the amount and type of fat. To understand the complex relationships between nutrition and chronic disease, we need to delve deeper into nutrition and understand how the nutrients interact with our body. Only then are we able to understand why some foods increase and others decrease the risk of chronic disease.

Calories Are Good for You

Many individuals shrink from calories and erroneously think they are bad. This is echoed by innumerable ads, which make us believe that calories are the enemy of beauty and good looks. Nothing is more misleading. In fact the first and foremost need of our body is the need for calories. Energy in our food, measured by the calorie unit (in Britain they use a different unit, which is called the joule), is absolutely necessary for growth during childhood survival and for good health in adults. In fact the energy in our food is life-giving, keeps our body machinery going, and allows us to engage in innumerable wonderful activities, such as hiking, playing tennis, seeing, and hearing. Even thinking requires energy. During sleep, when the body shuts down voluntary activities, we still require energy, mostly to keep our body temperature at a constant level and to drive our heartbeat and the muscles we use for breathing, as for the functioning of all other organs. Energy is absolutely necessary for survival; it allows us to be active and provides us with the stamina and zest for life. Next to water, energy is the most important nutritional requirement.

The need for energy varies from person to person and throughout life. During active growth more energy is needed. The newborn doubling his/her birth weight in a matter of months, for example, has a daily energy requirement per pound of body weight, which is three times higher than that of the adult. Energy need is also high during the adolescent growth spurt and during severe physical activity. Everybody needs energy to keep the body temperature at a constant level. Energy powers the cellular activity of body systems and also the physical activity we are engaged in. The sedentary person uses about two-thirds of food energy for body processes and one-third for activity. An extremely active person on the other hand uses a much greater amount of energy for activity. While the energy to keep our body systems going is the same from day to day, the energy for activity varies with our level of physical activity.

We have no control over the energy used by our organs and tissues, but we can voluntarily vary our activity level. Consequently we have some control over how much energy we require. Exercise helps burn calories and therefore all weight-reduction programs that call for increased activity in addition to reducing dietary calories are more effective than those that call for dieting alone. Individuals not on weight reduction who increase their activity can eat more food to allow a more varied diet.

A high-carbohydrate, low-fat diet along with exercise is the best means of preventing and treating obesity.
   —A. P. Simopoulos, "Nutritional Fitness:" A conference report. *Nutrition Today* 27 (1992): 24–29.

A person's energy requirement can be calculated, but it requires cumbersome methods and may be inaccurate (see Appendix B). The simplest and for most purposes entirely adequate method to check the adequacy of your energy intake is weighing yourself at regular intervals. If an adult's body weight is stable over a long period of time, he or she receives adequate calories from the diet to cover the body's need. Studies in which a person's energy intake is compared to the energy output are known as energy balance studies. During the adult years, with a stable body weight, the energy balance is zero, the dietary energy intake is the same as the energy output (Input = Output). During growth, children need extra energy for growth (Input must be greater than output). They become stunted if energy is limited. Only with optimum energy intakes from food can children grow optimally.

Energy Input

Just as foods vary in their vitamin, mineral, and protein content, so the foods we eat vary in their energy content. One ounce of dietary fat, for example, contains 250 (or 9 Cal per gram). One ounce of starch on the other hand contains only 112 (or 4 Cal per gram). One ounce of pure protein also contains 112 and provides the same amount of energy as starch (4 Cal per gram). The significant fact is that fats and oils are high-calorie sources, providing more than twice the amount of energy as do protein or starch on a weight for weight basis. All fats and oils are high-calorie sources. Solid fats like butter, margarine, or lard provide the same calories as olive oil, or sunflower oil, or the fat in beef and chicken (9 Cal per gram fat). The same is true for different carbohydrates, such as sugar, honey, or the starch in flour, bread, cereals, pasta, and potato. They all provide the same number of calories (4 Cal per gram). An exception is fiber, a complex carbohydrate, which is only partially broken down by the bacterial flora of the gut. It is believed that fiber may only provide a fraction of the energy of starch. The innumerable proteins too are equivalent in terms of calories and whether we get one gram of protein from an egg, beef, or milk, one gram of protein will always give us four calories of food energy.

Fats and oils are the most condensed energy sources in our diet. Weight for weight they provide more than twice as many calories as proteins and carbohydrates.

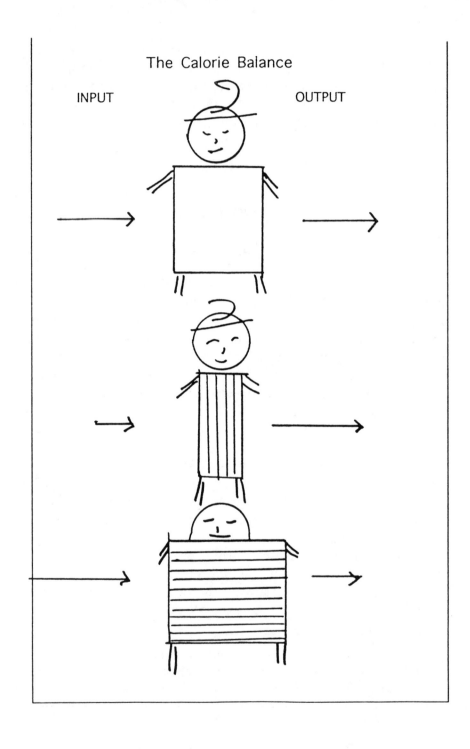

The measurement of food energy was one of the most brilliant discoveries made during the last century. If we were to burn one gram of sugar in a flame, for example, the energy liberated would be four Calories. Slow "burning" of one gram of sugar in the body also releases four Calories. In the body the slow burning in the presence of oxygen is a very controlled, step-wise process, which liberates the energy in tiny bursts. Our body behaves just like a machine. Fuel is necessary to make it go. Without fuel our body very soon would come to a standstill.

Besides the three classes of energy nutrients, we need to mention alcohol. Although not considered a nutrient, alcohol is the only other energy source for humans beside fat, carbohydrate, and protein. Alcohol has a caloric content intermediate between fat and sugar. It provides the body with approximately seven Calories per gram of alcohol. For example, a glass of wine with an alcohol content of 14 percent provides approximately 126 Cal, a twelve-ounce beer 148 Cal and an eight ounce highball cocktail 166 Cal. A slice of Hollywood bread in comparison provides 68 Cal.

Calories from our food (not from alcohol) should be our allies and not our enemies. Therefore it is advantageous to know which foods provide energy and how we expend the energy in activity. The more active a person is, the more calories his body burns. People who love to eat and are on the chubby side need to start moving and exercising. Any physical activity, such as walking, swimming, bicycling, is helpful. In addition review your diet for high-caloric foods and substitute those with similar tasty low-calorie items (see table 11).

Table 11

How Long It Takes to Use the Energy in Foods

Food	Cal	Walking	Running	Reclining
			In Minutes	
Apple	101	19	5	78
Cereal/milk	200	38	10	154
Doughnut	151	29	8	116
Bread/butter	78	15	4	60
Carrot, raw	42	8	2	32
Orange	68	13	4	52
Pancake/syrup	124	24	6	95
Peach	46	9	2	35
Pie/apple	377	73	19	290
Pizza	180	35	9	138
Pork chop	314	60	16	242
Potato chips	108	21	6	83
Hamburger	350	67	18	269
Club sandwich	590	113	30	454
Spaghetti	396	76	20	305
Steak	235	45	12	181
Shortcake	400	77	21	308
Ice cream	193	37	10	148

Nutrient Dense Is Desirable

Nutrient-dense foods contain liberal nutrients in relationship to calories. Such foods are good sources of vitamins and minerals and provide moderate numbers of calories. For example, whole-wheat and white bread provide the same energy. The former also contains a variety of B vitamins, minerals, and fiber;

the highly refined flour is low in these nutrients. Many other such examples could be cited. A comparison of molasses with sugar shows that sugar is practically devoid of nutrients while molasses is a source of iron and other trace minerals. Food processing may strip food of naturally present nutrients. Diets that include many highly processed foods are harder to balance because their nutrient density may have been reduced during processing.

A nutrient-dense food is a significant nutrient source in relation to the calories it provides.

A selection of foods with high-nutrient density is desirable for everybody but is especially critical for children during their growing years. When nutrients are limited, children's growth cannot proceed as it should. Eating diets with low nutrient density and a high proportion of calories may lead to obesity and the child at the same time is malnourished. Adults predisposed to obesity, adults who are small, and/or inactive, the elderly and dieters all need to be aware of selecting foods with high nutrient density.

Any diet with fewer than 1,200 Cal per day cannot provide all the vitamins and minerals in adequate amounts, even if nutrient dense foods are selected. Individuals on severe weight-reduction programs need to select foods with high nutrient density and in addition may require a vitamin/mineral supplement.

Empty Calories Are Fattening

A food devoid of nutrients but rich in calories is a food with empty calories. Table sugar provides empty calories. So do honey and many fats (except the oils, which contain the essential fatty acids, vitamins E and K). All alcoholic beverages provide empty calories although some wines may provide iron, and beer may provide some B vitamins. Some food combinations, such as a salad with olive oil, will result in a nutrient-dense food combination because of the vitamins and minerals in salad greens and tomatoes while the calories are derived from the oil in salad dressing.

An empty calorie food provides only calories without significant other nutrients, such as vitamins, minerals, protein, or fiber.

Calorie Counting: Not Worth the Trouble

A whole population of dieters count their daily calories for fear of eating diets with too many calories. Yet is calorie counting the answer to the problem? Calorie counting takes time and may be required for diets given for medical reasons. For weight-reduction programs, counting calories alone is not sufficient and even may be misleading. Calories are important but they are only a part. Eating foods with high-nutrient density and eliminating empty calories while increasing activity to burn stored body fat is the way to proceed. Such exercise and diet changes have multiple health benefits and encourge well-being. They are beneficial for our digestion; our circulatory system and general health improve. Overall, we feel better and we adjust to a lifestyle that is sustainable lifelong.

Step Six: Calories—More or Less?

Today we need to decide what kind of policy about calories each of us needs to pursue. We all need energy on a daily basis. If you are a person who can eat and eat but never gets fat, you can forget about calories as long as you eat a varied and balanced diet. But if you are a person who has a problem with the bulge, calories have to be chosen with care. Even in cases in which the obesity is a matter of our constitution, the selection of calories is critical. In most cases we have at least some control, and as long as we recognize the situation, we can do something about it.

Whatever your caloric needs are, you should start with the recommended servings from the food guide as we have discussed in previous sections. If you have no problem with obesity, include some servings from the fat/sugar group, preferably using soft fat or oils rather than fats that are hard at room temperature. Another way to add calories is by extra servings from the grain and vegetable group.

If your body-mass index tells you that you are approaching obesity or are in the obese range, you need to cut out *empty calories* as much as possible. *Above all, cut the calories from fats to the quick.* You do need some of the polyunsaturated fats, which you can obtain from vegetable oils and ocean fish. The foods to cross out are deep-fried foods, fatty meats of all kinds, high-fat dairy products, ice creams as well as foods to which fats were added during cooking or high-fat spreads. You need to start reading food labels and to familiarize yourself with the amount of fat and the total calories of the food you want to buy. Once you start on a regular exercise program, it is possible to increase your calories.

The reduction of fat in the diet can be felt acutely because fats give a pleasant taste to foods. This is where substitutions are a real boon. We don't need to cover a potato with sour cream. Add some herbs, such as basil with a dash of lemon and salt. Top spaghetti with smothered tomato cubes with a dash of pepper and salt, and if you wish, just a little olive oil. There are even recipes for excellent vegetarian pizzas! Instead of butter on your toast, use a good jam. Remove skin from chicken, and when you boil meat to make a stew, let it cool and skim off all the fat. Your food can be delicious without all the fat, but you need to reeducate yourself to cook and eat differently.

Fat is digested slowly and therefore fatty meals stay in your stomach longer than carbohydrate foods. If you reduce the fat in your diet, you lose some of the satiety value of your food and it becomes important that you have regular meals to prevent hunger episodes, which result in loss of appetite control. Fiber that is low in calories and has the property of expanding to hold water will counteract some of the loss of satiety value experienced with low-fat diets. To get adjusted, distribute your food throughout the day and have some of your daily food ready during a time when hunger strikes. Some people are better than others in coping with their hunger feelings. A glass of water may dull the hunger for a while for some, but others need to have something more substantial. Not being prepared for the eventuality of a hunger episode means that the food-seeking behavior takes over and you will feast surreptitiously, perhaps on Twinkies, or on a chocolate bar just before a meal. Well-spaced meal patterns are least likely to encourage this.

If you have identified what will work for you, prepare some cycle menus for a while until you have adjusted to the new diet pattern. Simply follow strictly the recommended servings and make sure that you get the proper serving sizes. Cycle menus are a set of daily meal plans in which everything is planned ahead. To plan all meals for a week take time, but soon you will get experience and your program becomes almost automatic.

More thought is required for people living in a family with individuals requiring vastly different daily calories. For example, the husband may be underweight and the wife obese or vice versa. Eating exactly the same meals is problematic for both. Again, if you start with a low-fat diet, which is varied and balanced, you can make the adjustments to the food for the underweight or extremely active person. One way is to provide double portions of grains and vegetables for an extremely active person. Another is to include somewhat more empty calories, or provide nutritious snacks between meals. Let the person's food preference and body weight be the guide.

The relationship of exercise to our calorie requirement is profoundly important. Exercise as part of a healthy lifestyle provides an important benefit in that we can include more calories in our basic food plan. Exercise is also a must during weight-reduction programs since this will increase our energy expenditure and burn extra calories. During a weight-reduction program, we want to protect our muscles and ideally only reduce our body fat. Therefore, only food calories should decrease—not any of the other nutrients—with the simultaneous increase of our energy expenditure through exercise.

Specifics to Do

1. Use your body weight (in pounds) and height (in inches) to determine your body-mass index (see Appendix F). Record whether you fall in the normal, underweight, or overweight range.

2. Plan your diet using the recommended servings from the food groups.

3. If you are underweight, increase your food intake from the cereal, vegetable, and fruit group and add two or three more servings from the meat group. You also can include some items from the sugar/fat group.

4. If your BMI is in the obese range or very close to it, stick to the recommended servings. Make sure you include some protein with every meal and distribute your food throughout the day so that you do not feel hungry. If you lead a sedentary life, start walking to get your circulation going. Find out what determines your mind-set and works against you.

5. Check your body weight and record any changes. Check your BMI at regular intervals to document your progress.

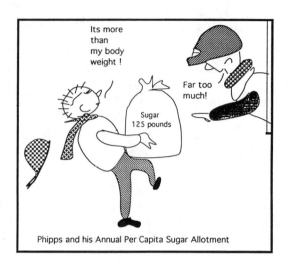

Phipps and his Annual Per Capita Sugar Allotment

Chapter VIII
Carbos for Energy

Carbohydrates are the major source of energy for our body; therefore it is vital to know which foods provide them. Dietary carbohydrates include sugars, starch, and fiber and come from a variety of food sources. All of them, except milk sugar (lactose) and traces of animal starch in meat and liver (glycogen), are plant products. Carbohydrates provide us with 4 Cal per gram (or 112 Cal per oz). As already mentioned, fiber is an exception; it is not digested by our gut enzymes but is partially broken down by the action of bacteria in our large intestine. The exact caloric contribution of fiber is not known. Researchers suggest that fiber, weight for weight, provides only a small fraction of the calories of starch.

Sweet Sugars

Sugars in our diets come from ripe fruits, honey, molasses, syrups, and table sugar. Sugars and corn syrup are added to innumerable products, such as beverages, sweets, cereals, cookies, and desserts. Many foods contain hidden sugar, such as tomato paste and Hamburger Helper. All sugars taste sweet, some more than others. Fructose in honey and ripe fruits and common table sugar are the sweetest sugars, while glucose tastes less sweet and milk sugar even less. Dietary sugars are rapidly absorbed from the gut into the blood, and all are converted to glucose. Glucose, the blood sugar, is taken up by brain, muscle, and liver and other cells. Inside the cell, the glucose is broken down to release its energy, which is used for muscle contraction, brain function, and building new tissue among many other functions. Because the sugars need little digestion, they are called simple carbohydrates.

Starchy Foods—Staples the World Over

Starch is a complex carbohydrate because it is made up of glucose particles chained together forming treelike, rather large granules. Plants store starch in grains, seeds, tubers, and many other plant structures. Grains of wheat, rice, corn, barley, sorghum, millet, oats, rye and buckwheat are the staples in diets around the world because of their high starch content. Starch is also the main component of potatoes, yams, sweet potatoes, and the less known taro and topinambur and occurs in many vegetables and fruits. When starch-containing foods are eaten, the starch must be digested. The glucose liberated from starch during digestion enters the blood and joins the blood glucose pool.

Whole grains are important sources of dietary fiber, trace minerals, several vitamins, and other compounds of interest in disease prevention, including phyto-estrogens and antioxidants. *Whole grains* are furthermore low in fat and contain no cholesterol. A consensus conference held in 1993 suggests that of the six to eleven servings of the bread, cereal, rice, and pasta group, three should be *whole-grain servings.*

—J. L. Slavin, "Whole Grains and Health," *Nutrition Today* 29 (1994): 6–11.

Fiber Too Tough for Digestion

Fiber is a mixture of complex carboydrates, which in recent years has achieved notoriety because low-fiber diets have been linked to chronic disease. Fibers are not digested by our digestive juices but stay in the gut and by attracting water increase stool mass and help prevent constipation. The function of the different fibers, such as cellulose and pectin, is under intense investigation. Much is still to be learned, but we know that in addition to preventing constipation, fiber can protect us from certain cancers, enhance cholesterol excretion in bile, and help better blood glucose regulation in diabetics. Bacteria partially break down fiber in the colon, and it is believed that the breakdown products increase gut activity. Unfortunately studies with fiber have often given controversial results, probably because fibers are not well defined, and because different fibers act differently—for example, data indicate that only soluble fiber, such as fiber from apple, oat bran, or orange, reduces blood-cholesterol levels while fibers from wheat and corn bran are inactive in this respect. All fibers are beneficial for digestion.

Cellulose—insoluble fiber—we get from whole wheat, bran, the cabbage family, peas and beans, apples and root vegetables.

Pectin and gums—soluble fiber—we get from apple, citrus fruits, strawberries, oatmeal, also from dried beans and other legumes.

Carbohydrates with Each Meal

At least half of our calories should come from carbohydrates but preferably somewhat more. This means that carbohydrate-rich foods should make up a major portion of our diet and therefore need to be included with every meal. With the great number of grains, breads, cereals, pasta, and tubers, it is no problem to select for variety.

While weight-for-weight starch and sugar provide equal amounts of calories, there are strong health reasons to minimize the dietary intake of sugar. Sugar in sweets, a source of empty concentrated calories, is in large part responsible for tooth decay. A hefty dose of sugar will stimulate the release of excess insulin, the hormone that facilitates glucose uptake to convert it into fat. After a sugar load, your blood sugar may rise extraordinarily high and then plummet below normal to produce intense sugar craving. Sugars from all kinds of fruits and a small amount of table sugar used as a flavoring agent can be part of our diets, but the major portion of carbohydrate energy should come from complex carbohydrates, such as grains, tubers, and their products. To prevent excessive sugar intake, we need constantly to be on the alert and read labels on cereals and other items for their added sugar, fructose, sucrose, or syrup content.

We have a wide selection of dietary complex carbohydrates to choose from. The one point to keep in mind is to include enough fiber from whole grains. Individuals have different tolerances for fiber, and each needs to find his own level of intake that allows regular bowel evacuation without getting diarrhea. In addition to cereals, vegetables such as carrots, broccoli, cabbage, celery, legumes, and fruits contribute fiber to our daily diets. No single food source is sufficient to provide the amount of fiber beneficial to our health. A daily intake of between twenty and thirty grams of dietary fiber from vegetables, fruits, and grain products has been recommended. This amount may be unrealistically high for low-calorie diets. A more realistic recommendation is to get at least one gram fiber per one hundred Cal (see figure 7).

The "Right Kinds" of Carbohydrates

How our body uses carbohydrate foods is a fascinating story. Much of it is known while much we still do not yet understand—such as the heuristic effect of sugar, for example. We like the taste of sugar because it gives us pleasure and makes us feel good. But why sugar specifically and not some other dietary constituent, such as broccoli? And why is it that some individuals after repeatedly eating sweets get addicted to sugar while others don't? Once one is addicted to sugar, undesirable consequences can follow, and it is difficult to break out of this cycle of sugar craving. Eating regular meals and a nutritious, mixed diet that is satisfying is the first step in breaking the cycle, but sometimes professional help is needed.

All dietary sugars and starches we use for energy end up as blood glucose. If we eat carbohydrates as part of a mixed diet, together with protein and some fat, the absorption of glucose from the gut is slow so that blood glucose is not overwhelmed. If, on the other hand, we eat a high sugar load, the glucose enters the bloodstream so rapidly that very high blood glucose levels are

Nutrition Facts

Serving Size ½ cup (114g)
Servings Per Container 4

Amount Per Serving

Calories 90   Calories from Fat 30

% Daily Value*

Total Fat 3g	5%
Saturated Fat 0g	0%
Cholesterol 0mg	0%
Sodium 300mg	13%
Total Carbohydrate 13g	4%
Dietary Fiber 3g	12%
Sugars 3g	
Protein 3g	

Figure 7

produced. Such high swings in blood glucose may, over time, lead to diabetes. The dietary sugar load may stimulate insulin release from the pancreas so strongly that glucose is shunted into cells exceedingly rapidly. During such an episode, glucose is made rapidly into fat and the blood sugar drops to dangerously low levels. During low blood sugar (hypoglycemia), a person feels faint and trembling and in severe cases may pass out. The reason is that our brain uses only one energy source and this is glucose, not fat or protein. It seems rather paradoxical that eating a high sugar load actually results in low blood sugar. Treatment and prevention of hypoglycemia consists of eating a varied, low-sugar diet with adequate amounts of protein. Protein rescues the situation because some is slowly converted to glucose between meals, which prevents episodes of low blood sugar. Diet-related diabetes mellitus (type II) is often associated with obesity in individuals who consume empty-calorie and high-sugar diets. Eating a variety of foods that are nutrient dense, low in sugar, and adequate in fiber goes a long way to prevent problems related to faulty carbohydrate diets.

Step Seven: Carbos for Energy and Good Health

Three points need to be remembered about the carbohydrates in your diets: *Reduce sugar, increase fiber, use whole unrefined carbohydrate foods as the main source of daily calories.*

To make certain that sugar intake does not get out of hand, the contents of the sugar bowl should be used only sparingly. This is comparatively easy. More difficult is to limit the hidden sugar in foods. Sugar as a preservative prevents bacterial growth and for this reason it is added to many foods, such as jams and jellies and even to pickles. Other sources of sugar in our diets are soft drinks and syrup-packed fruits. One can of a soft drink for example may contain as many as five heaped teaspoons of sugar. Cereals that contain added sugar must be labeled for their sugar content. Reading food labels is a must in the selection of low sugar products.

EFFECT OF REPEATED HIGH
DIETARY SUGAR INTAKES ON BLOOD SUGAR

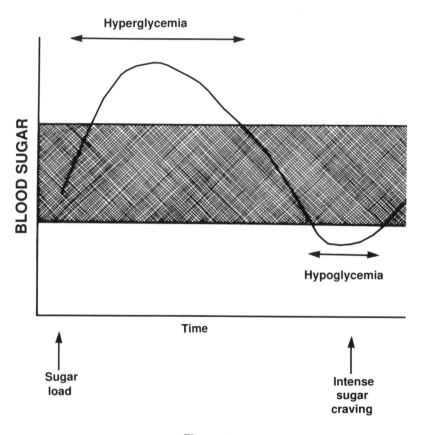

Figure 8

If you eat a variety of servings of vegetables and fruits as indicated in your diet plan, you already get a considerable amount of fiber. If in addition you select some whole grain cereals and breads that have a high fiber content to eat, with an occasional legume for your main meal, your dietary fiber intake will be adequate. Just by following the recommended basic meal plan, you will take care of your fiber. Fiber without sufficient fluid intake can lead to constipation. Make sure you drink fluid with your fiber foods to get the maximum benefit. Of course we can get fiber from supplements, and no doubt their occasional use has a place in the armament of home remedies. But since different food fibers seem to have unique effects, a mixture of vegetable, fruit, and grain fibers is most desirable. Furthermore, fiber needs to be part of our diet on a regular basis to get long-term effects.

We need to reeducate ourselves from the error of the older generation, which labored under the assumption that starchy foods are fattening. Today a balanced diet should contain more than half the calories from grains, cereals, breads, pasta, tubers like potatoes, legumes, fruits, and vegetables. It is often the added fat and sugar that are responsible for the "fattening." Butter on whole bread, sour cream on potato, fat on spaghetti, sugar added to cereals, the sugar and fat added to baked goods, all make high-calorie items out of low-calorie grain products. As a quick reference, you should get six servings of the grain group on the lowest calorie diet and up to eleven servings of grains on the high-calorie diet per day. As already mentioned before, the answer is not to cut out the starchy foods but to use them as part of the total diet. The fat traditionally used to give flavor to some of the grain foods can be replaced by a variety of herbs, spices, and tasty food combinations that are low-calorie items.

Specifics to Do

1. Check the distribution of carbohydrate foods in your meals. On the low-calorie diet, you should get at least six servings from the grain group. If you follow a three-meal plan, make sure you get two servings of

100

the grain/bread/pasta group at breakfast, lunch, and at supper. The number of servings of the grain, cereal/bread/pasta group depends on your energy need, but even with a low-calorie diet at least six servings per day are required.

2. As a start, select half of your grain/bread/pasta servings as whole-grain products with high fiber content. Increase or decrease this amount dependng on your need.

3. Read labels for sugar and dietary fiber content. Select items with low sugar and high fiber content.

4. For at least one day, write down how much total sugar in grams you get from your diet. If you get more than thirty grams (about one ounce) of sugar per day (more than 120 empty Cals), find out which foods contribute high sugar amounts. Try to limit some.

5. Write down also how much fiber you get from your daily food. Any food giving you more than 15 percent of the daily value is a good fiber source.

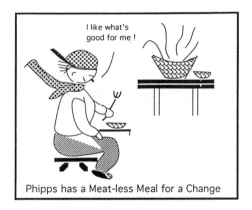

Phipps has a Meat-less Meal for a Change

Chapter IX
Your Protein Needs

Women's preoccupation often relates to calories, while men frequently are more concerned with protein because of muscle building. We all need a daily source of dietary protein. It is vital for our survival since every living cell in our body requires it. Proteins perform innumerable functions. Insulin regulates blood glucose, immune proteins fight infections, muscle protein fibers contract and allow us to move about, just to mention a few. The hundreds of unique proteins in our body are possible because they are made up of smaller units, the amino acids, which are arranged in varied patterns containing from a few to many thousands of these building blocks.

How Much Protein Is Enough?

The daily protein recommendation has slightly varied over the years. Approximately 50 g protein per day are recommended for women and sixty for men. Sometimes the daily protein need is calculated from our body weight (multiply lbs weight by 0.4). A 130-lb adult would then need 52 g of protein per day. (Do not use this method if you are extremely under- or overweight, which respectively under- or overestimates your protein need.) More protein is needed for growth, especially during the adolescent years, or during pregnancy (add another 11 g per day), and by lactating women (add up to 15 g per day). Vegetable proteins are required in slightly higher daily amounts (multiply body weight by 0.5 g protein).

Okay Protein Foods

Chicken, turkey, lean beef, veal, pork, lamb, fish, shellfish, egg white, wild game, rabbit, pheasant, venison, meatless low-fat combination dishes

---

The Energy in Proteins

All dietary proteins provide energy to the body (112 Cal per oz or 4 Cal per gram protein). But only approximately 10 to 15 percent of our daily energy requirement comes from protein (the majority is from carbohydrates and fat). When protein is used for energy, it is only partially broken down and the end product, urea, must be excreted by the kidney. The greater the consumption of protein, the more urea our kidneys must excrete. High-protein meals make people thirsty because more fluid is required for the excretion of the urea.

A gram is a unit of weight in the metric system. An ounce is about thirty grams.

Protein Foods Are Problematic

Although animal foods are excellent sources of a high quality protein, red meats and meat products are a significant source of saturated fat, which contributes to the risk of heart disease. Similarly, the protein in milk and cheese is a high-quality protein, but again the type of fat in dairy products is a problem. Egg contains an excellent protein, but egg yolk is the highest source of cholesterol in our diets. In addition, additives such as salt, nitrates, and others occur in ham, bacon, cold cuts, pickled meats, hot dogs, and sausages.

Meats with Too Much Fat or Salt

**"Prime" or heavily marbled and fatty meats
short ribs, spare ribs, fatty steak,
corned beef, pastrami, regular hamburger,
sausage, bacon, high-fat luncheon meat**

Because of the saturated fat, cholesterol, and salt in some of the protein foods of animal origin, it is wise to replace part of our

104

dietary animal protein with a vegetable protein source. Many individuals have even switched to completely vegetarian diets. To obtain adequate protein for the body's many functions, strict vegetarians—the vegans—must complement their protein.

Complementing Makes for Quality

Proteins from animal and plant food all contain the same twenty or so amino acids, although in different amounts and proportions. During the digestive process, the dietary proteins are broken down to free the amino acids. After they are absorbed into the circulation and taken up by our body cells, they are used to make our own protein. In fact, our cells are complex protein factories, and as long as we have the amino acids in sufficient amounts and favorable combinations, we are able to make all the proteins our body needs.

Our cells can make our protein in a highly efficient manner when we eat mixed diets that contain some protein-rich foods from animal sources, such as milk, egg, meats of all kinds, and fish. Animal proteins provide the amino acids in the most favorable amounts and proportions and therefore are called complete or high quality proteins. Plants that contain significant amounts of protein, such as grains, nuts, and legumes, provide amino-acid mixtures that are low in one or several amino acids. Such proteins are called incomplete or of low quality. Plant proteins are improved by mixing complementary proteins from two different plant sources. A meal of corn and beans, rice and soybeans or lentils, wheat and chickpeas provides high-quality protein because the two different protein sources complement each other. Grains have a shortage of the amino acid lysine found in liberal amounts in beans and soybeans. Conversely the sulphur amino acids are low in soybeans but abundant in cereal grains.

If you eat a mixed diet, as suggested by the Food Guide, you do not need to plan menus with complementary proteins. It only becomes an issue if you want to follow a strict vegetarian (vegan) diet. Many traditional vegetarian food combinations have evolved with complementary proteins to improve quality. Mexican recipes for corn products and beans, Chinese rice dishes with fermented soybean products such as tempe, or Indian wheat dishes eaten together with lentils are good examples of food mixtures with improved protein quality. The combination of the two proteins is superior to its parts. Healthy adults eating mixed or vegetarian diets usually receive more than enough protein. Children, on the other hand, need a source of animal protein for growth; otherwise they may become growth stunted.

Protein Combos for Meatless Meals

Grains and beans
Rice and tofu
Rice and lentils
Bread and peanut butter
Beans and taco
Macaroni and low-fat cheese
Cereals and milk
Bread and cheese
Potato and cultured milk

The American Protein Glut

The major thrust of the new food guide is to encourage vegetables and fruits and to deemphasize fatty meats. You might wonder whether such diets provide us with enough protein. To settle this question, study carefully the diet below, which is based on the food guide (the low-calorie diet, table 12). The diet provides 6 servings from the grain, 3 from the vegetable, 3 fruit, 2.5 milk, and 5 servings from the meat group. In the last column, the amount of protein for each food is given, and the protein for each meal calculated. At the end the total protein for this diet is given. *Total Protein for the Day: 83 Grams—More than Enough!* Note also that the major source of protein in this diet is chicken and milk, but the grain group and legumes are also a significant source while vegetables and fruits provide very little. Note also that the distribution of protein throughout the day is acceptable since some protein foods are eaten with every meal. This prevents excessive hunger and combats feelings of tiredness in between meals. The sample also shows that we get considerable protein

Table 12

Sample Diet

Meal	Food		(grams) Protein
Breakfast	Corn flakes	1/2 cup	0.9
	Milk 1%	1/2 cup	4.0
	Orange juice	6 oz	1.2
	Total for breakfast		*6.1*
Lunch	Chicken breast	3 oz	26.4
	Whole-wheat bread	2 slices	7.4
	Lettuce, chopped	1/2 cup	0.4
	Banana	1/2	0.6
	Total for lunch		*34.8*
Supper	Rice white	1 cup	5.5
	Kidney beans	0.5 cup	6.7
	Carrots	0.5 cup	0.8
	Broccoli	0.5 cups	2.3
	Egg, hard boiled	1 medium	6.3
	Apple	1 medium	0.3
	Total for supper		*21.9*
Late night snack	Lowfat yogurt	1 cup	11.9
	Saltine crackers	4 each	1.1
	Cheddar cheese	1 oz	7.1
	Total for snacks		*20.0*

(twenty grams) from snacks, although in this sample it would have been better to have a snack at midmorning rather than in the night. No beverages were included in this analysis because coffee, tea, seltzer, etc., do not provide protein.

The sample diet given above is a low-calorie diet (1,429 Cal). Individuals who have higher energy requirements may need as many as seven meat and eleven grain servings per day instead of the five meat and six grains, as in the sample above. Such diets would provide 30 g more protein, with a total daily intake of 114 g protein. A truly luxury intake! The protein would also be sufficient if you were to omit beef and chicken completely and instead to select a second serving of beans, and two servings of peanut butter. The upshot is that by eating according to the food guide even on extremely low-calorie mixed diets, adults get more than enough protein per day.

Watch Protein Foods on Tight Budgets

Meats, fish, chicken, turkey, milk, cheese, and eggs are expensive items on the shopping list. For those who must budget, it is good to know that some of the less expensive meat cuts can be nutritionally excellent because of less fat content. Chicken, which usually contains less fat than beef, often is on sale and can be kept frozen until used. Fish, an excellent source of protein, quite low in fat, is usually expensive, but tuna packed in water is one of the least expensive protein sources, good for sandwiches, casseroles, and other recipes. Pound for pound, cold cuts and sausages are usually more expensive than chicken, and they are often high in fat and salt. Turkey and chicken parts can be used inexpensively for delicious soups and stews. Combination dishes such as beans and corn, lentils and rice, soybeans and pasta are less expensive meat substitutes.

Amino Acid Supplements Are a Waste

The use of amino acid supplements has become a craze among muscle builders. These items are practically useless because the protein in a small piece of chicken, fish, or in a good vegetable protein source provides amino acids in equal or greater amounts and superior proportions. Food protein is cheaper, providing actually more protein in a healthier form. Furthermore, single amino acids taken in pills are dangerous because they produce amino acid imbalances in the body, which are detrimental to health. It is well known, for example, that one amino acid in excess without all the other amino acids can induce a protein deficiency in the brain, the consequences of which are not well known.

Muscle Loss during Fasting

During fasting, or during too severe weight reduction, our body protein is used excessively for energy. Muscle breaks down and the amino acids freed are made into glucose to use as an energy source for our heart, breathing muscles, and the brain. This is one of the reasons why starvation diets should not be used for weight reduction. Better weight-reduction diets provide all the nutrients including protein and *only reduce calories below the daily calorie need to protect our muscle mass.* Weight-reduction programs that increase physical activity and moderately decrease dietary calories encourage the breakdown of the fat stored in our adipose tissue rather than our muscles.

Step Eight: Your Protein Check

If you eat the five to six servings (remember one ounce of meat is one serving) of foods from the meat group as suggested and the two to three servings from the dairy group, you will automatically receive enough protein to cover your daily need. Pregnant women, the elderly, and children during the adolescent growth spurt will need somewhat more protein to cover their respective special demands. The U.S. population in general has no problem with their protein and even junk foods (not recommended), and fast foods usually provide sufficient protein. There are, of course, individuals whose protein nutrition is problematic, but these are usually sick people, those who have gastrointestinal problems, also alcoholics whose gut is wrecked by alcohol, or the elderly who eat very limited diets, or individuals suffering from anorexia nervosa.

The problem with protein foods is their fat content. The only really important points we need to consider are the amount of fat in meats and dairy foods and the high salt content of processed meats. We can help ourselves to control these factors by buying lean meats and by trimming the fat before cooking. Use a cooking method that requires no added fat. Use non-stick pans and if you need some fat to prevent sticking to the pan, apply some with a brush. There are many ways to be creative. When you buy cold-cut meats, be careful to choose the least processed and the least salty—such as sliced roast beef or turkey breast.

The dairy group is also an excellent source of high-quality protein in our diet. Again the fat in milk is the problem. Use low-fat milks. If you are on a tight budget, you can stretch your milk by mixing 2 percent fat milk and an equal amount of reconstituted milk from non-fat dry powder to give a 1 percent fat product. Milk, yogurt, and cottage cheese are labeled in terms of their fat content. Cheeses with unknown fat content can be a problem. Select hard cheeses, which usually contain less fat. Use spreads and soft cheese sparingly.

To Do

1. Check your diet for the number of servings from the meat group and the milk/dairy group. This will give you a quick reference whether you get adequate, too little or liberal protein in your diet. If your diet excludes whole food groups, such as the meat and/or dairy group, your protein may be compromised. If you

110

are a vegan—a strict vegetarian—you need to use recipes in which complementary proteins are mixed. If you get too many servings from the meat and dairy group, you may get too much of the wrong kind of fat. In the latter case, substitute legumes for some of the beef and meat servings.

2. Educate yourself to choose the correct portion sizes. One ounce of lean meat (approximately thirty grams) is one portion. A three-ounce piece of meat, chicken, or fish for lunch and two portions of meat substitute for supper will provide sufficient protein. Include a serving from the dairy group for breakfast and possibly a snack. For balance have a protein food from the dairy or the meat group with each meal.

3. Note the fat content of your servings from the dairy group. Select low-fat products. It is hard to go from one extreme to another. If you are used to whole milk, go to 2 percent and gradually decrease to 1 percent milk.

4. Observe whether or not you get the recommended servings from the dairy group. If you have a problem with overweight, select dairy products and meats with the very lowest fat content.

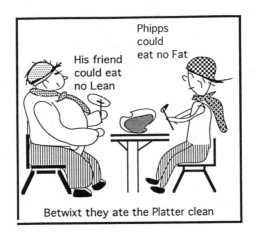

His friend
could eat
no Lean

Phipps
could
eat no Fat

Betwixt they ate the Platter clean

Chapter X

Fats:
Prevent Trouble—
Get Their Benefit

Fat is the most concentrated source of energy in our diet. Weight for weight it provides more than twice the calories of protein and carbohydrate, and high fat diets contribute significantly to obesity. Our body stores fat when the calories in our diet exceed the energy need for our body machinery and daily activities. Under such conditions dietary fat as well as fat that is formed from excess dietary carbohydrate and protein is deposited in fat cells of adipose tissue. Warehouses of fat, the fat cells are located under our skin and around body organs. They slowly fill up and once they are full, the fat stubbornly wants to stay there. Only during energy shortages, as during exercise, or when we eat low-calorie diets is our warehouse fat mobilized and used to cover our energy needs.

"Fat Chance: Obesity Is in the Genes!" writes *U.S. News* on December 12, 1994.
    But take heart: turn to flab-reducing lifestyles!

Everybody needs body fat stores for good health. Adult women require somewhat more than men. However, with increasing fat accumulation, overweight and eventually obesity develop. Obesity predisposes a person to health problems, which can become life threatening. Apart from energy storage, body fat has other vital functions. Our brain, for example, is extremely rich in structural fatlike substances (lipids); breakdown products of fats provide building blocks for hormones, such as the sex hormones; and the fat from oils and ocean fish forms prostaglandins, which are hormones required for smooth muscle contraction, acid production of the stomach, uterine contraction during birth, and for proper immune function.

Unfortunately people in modern affluent societies with abundant food high in calories often eat too much fat and fat of the wrong kind. No other nutrient class is so intimately associated with chronic disease as excess dietary fat. Perfectly healthy people by eating too much, and the wrong kind of fat, may become prone to obesity, heart disease, stroke, gallbladder disease, and even some cancers. Selecting diets with moderate fat content and a balance of the various types of fat can reduce the risk and likelihood of suffering chronic diseases.

Table 13

More Jiggle Than Ever*

Americans aged 20–74,
who are overweight

1960–62	24.3%
1971–74	25.0%
1988–91	33.3%

*Tracy Watson, "What Really Plumps You Up," *U.S. News and World Report*, December 12, 1994, reprinted by permission.

Supercharged with Calories

When fats and oils are broken down in our body, they release a burst of energy. Each gram of fat or oil releases nine calories. Dietary fat not used immediately for our daily energy need is deposited in adipose tissues. Overloading our diets with energy-rich foods over some period of time results in overweight and eventually in obesity, a problem for many Americans. Yet diet is not the only culprit. Our genes, our hormones, our modern lifestyle, psychological problems, and our sedentary lifestyle with too little activity coupled with high-fat diets all contribute to obesity.

The solution for flabby bodies lies in the old mantra: more exercise, less high-calorie food.

Once obesity has developed over a period of time, it usually requires an heroic effort to mobilize the fat from adipose tissue. Even if an obese person successfully has lost some of the stored fat, the remaining empty fat cells become hypersensitive. They practically crave fat, and the moment the person eats fat and other high caloric foods, the fat cells fill up with a vengeance. The yoyo effect of multiple weight reduction periods followed by remissions seems just as detrimental to health as the steady state of obesity. Since we cannot change our genes (yet) and have little influence on our hormones, the only armament to combat obesity is a change in lifestyle. Three things are paramount:

1. *Find out and remedy what sets off your uncontrollable eating pattern.*
2. *Choose diets that are adequate in nutrients but low in calories, especially from fat (and alcohol).*
3. *Increase your daily calorie expenditure through activity.*

The Mixed Bag of Fats

A confusing issue is the fact that fats and oils are always mixtures of several types of fats. Therefore we need to know something about their makeup since different types interact with our body in very different ways. From a practical standpoint, we need to know only three groups of fats. The *saturated fats* are solid at room temperature; they predominate in butter, beef, pork, and in some of the tropical seed oils from coconut and palm kernels. When oils are fully hydrogenated, as corn oil in some vegetable shortenings, the oils are converted to solid, saturated fats. A fully saturated fat carries the maximum number of hydrogen atoms, and therefore the fat cannot react with the oxygen in air. Such fats do not get rancid, are stable in heat, and are popular in recipes in which the fat is heated as in deep frying. However, the saturated fats are the culprits as far as disease is concerned, and their use in modern diets needs to be monitored and limited.

All dietary fats and oils are mixtures of saturated, monounsaturated, and polyunsaturated fats.

The second group of fats are the *polyunsaturated fats,* which are liquid or semisolid at room temperature. This group of fats predominate in corn-, cottonseed-, safflower-, soybean-, sunflower-, sesame seed-, and canola oil. They are also found in ocean fish, like salmon, herring, and sardines, and some of the oils in nuts. Because these fats have multiple sites with missing hydrogen atoms that allow interaction, they are affected by heat and air and easily get rancid. Rancidity in oils can be prevented by storing them at low temperature and in air-tight containers. (Most oils contain vitamin E, the natural antioxidant that keeps the oil from becoming rancid.) The dietary intake of polyunsaturated fats in general is low in many American diets. This is a concern because they protect from atherosclerosis. Their dietary intake should be encouraged while at the same time total fat and saturated fat intake should decrease.

The third group of fats are the *monounsaturated fats* of which olive oil and the fat in avocado are good sources. They are intermediate between the saturates and polyunsaturates. They appear to have a positive health benefit but are still under intense investigation.

Fats for a Healthy Heart

Selecting fats and oils from the many products offered in supermarkets is a formidable undertaking. Should I use margarine or butter, hot or cold pressed olive oil, corn or sunflower oil, or any of the other fats and oils? The same confusing variety of oils is also found in salad dressing and mayonnaise, not to mention the different types of fats in meats, poultry, sausages, and cold cuts. How can we take into account the different kinds and amounts of fat in all these products?

To select fats and oils, we need to keep in mind the three types of fats (the saturates, polyunsaturates, and the monounsaturates—sometimes called the saturates, polys, and monos) and also remember that all fats are mixtures of the three types but that usually one of the types predominates. As figure 9 shows, the fat with the highest proportion of saturates is coconut fat. The other major saturated fats are butterfat, beef fat and palm oil. Diets that provide a great deal of these fats contain overall too much saturated fat. Chicken and turkey to a lesser extent also contain saturates, but most of the fat in these foods is in the skin, which can be easily removed.

All the fats given in the table contain some monounsaturated fats, with olive oil leading (contains approximately 80 percent). Good sources of monos are also pecan and almonds and several other nuts. On the other end of the spectrum is coconut fat, with hardly any monos. Scientists have thought that the monos were so to speak neutral in their relation to health, but recently new data indicate that they may have a beneficial effect. However, we always need to remember that all fats and oils are high calorie sources and can contribute to obesity.

Positive effects in preventing atherosclerosis are observed with the polyunsaturates. Corn oil, sunflower, soybean, and safflower oils contain significant amounts of polys. Lesser, but still significant amounts are also found in nuts such as pecans, peanuts, and almonds. A special type of polyunsaturates (scientists call them the omega-3 fats) occurs in ocean fish, and to a lesser extent in soybean, and canola oil. The inclusion in our diets of such fats is highly beneficial. The omega-3 polys not only protect us from high blood cholesterol (hypercholesterolemia) but also affect our blood-clotting mechanism and reduce the chance of a heart attack due to blood clot formation.

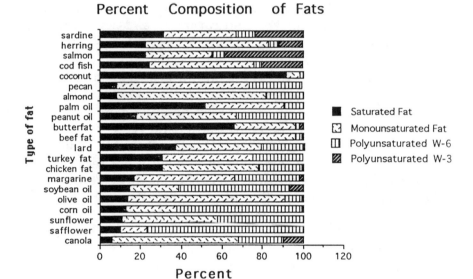

Figure 9

Omega-3 Fats Affect Cardiovascular Disease

by: prevention of platelet aggregation
decreasing blood clotting
dissolving blood clots
decreasing mild hypertension
decreasing blood viscosity.

—Alexander Leaf, M.D., *Nutrition Reviews*
50 (5) (1992): 150–152.

While the polys of oils are desirable, a controversy has arisen about oils that have been altered by the process of hydrogenation. In order to make a polyunsaturated oil more solid so that it can be used as a spread, hydrogens are introduced into the polys by an industrial process to form *partially hydrogenated fats.* Unfortunately during this process, an unusual type of fat (fat which contains trans-fatty acids) is produced in small but significant amounts. Data suggested in the past that these were may be harmless. Recent studies, however, indicate that they may contribute to heart disease as do saturated fats. Partially hydrogenated fats are now under intense investigation in relation to health. From a practical standpoint, it is possible to identify these types of fats in food products by reading food labels. Any food containing *partially* hydrogenated oils or fat may contain some trans-fatty acids. Future research will need to define their exact effects on health.

That the amount of total fat and the type of fat in our diet is important in preventing disease has been shown in many studies around the globe. Scientific debate still rages about some points related to the types of fat. We still have gaps in our knowledge, and this makes it difficult to formulate what the "ideal diet" should be, but from the extensive knowledge accrued, it is possible today to formulate diets with low risks for heart disease. It is quite clear that too many butterballs, coconut, and beef drippings aren't good for us. This does not mean that we need to exclude all these fats but that we need to use them sparingly. First, cut down on total fat intake by selecting meat with the least fat, trimming meats before cooking, and choosing cooking methods that require the least added fat. Second, select low-fat dairy products. Use milk with 1 percent milkfat rather than whole milk. Read labels for fat content when you buy dairy products, including cheeses and ice cream. Also look for hidden sources of fats, such as in dressings, mayonnaise, baked goods, even crackers, etc. The third point is to strike a balance between the three different types of fats. Substitute oils whenever possible for solid fat, and include both types of polys, those from vegetable oils and those from fish. And remember: get ocean fish rather than fresh-water fish. Fresh-water fish does not contain significant amounts of the omega-3 fats.

A good daily balance of the three types of fat has been suggested as providing one-third saturates, one-third monos, and one-third polys. On a daily basis, this is difficult to achieve since the amounts and types of fats vary from day to day, depending on the composition of the meals you choose. Keeping total fat low and substituting oils for some solid fats, are important steps for good health.

American children older than three years of age already show signs of fatty streaks in their arteries and higher blood cholesterol than children in countries with lower saturated fat intakes.
> **—L. Snetselaar, R.M. Lauer, "Childhood Diet and the Atherosclerotic Process,"**
> ***Nutrition Today* 27(1) (1992): 22–28.**

Good or Bad Fats—Good or Bad Foods?

We often talk as if some foods are bad and others good. "Eat carrots; they are good for your eyes," or "Don't eat butter; it is bad for your heart!" Such statements, which convey the idea that some foods are either good or bad, are completely erroneous. Foods are neither good nor bad per se (except if they have been spoiled by bacterial contamination). But a food can be used the wrong or the right way. It is entirely a matter of balance. Some sugar as a sweetener is all right, but lots of sugar in our diet will provide too many empty calories. Some fiber in the diet is good for our digestion, but too much fiber can make a person miserable with internal rumblings. Some saturated fats are desirable to provide us with energy, but too much will overload our system. This is equally true for the polyunsaturated fat; some is beneficial but too much may also lead to problems.

For every food and every nutrient, we have optimal intakes. Too much or too little is undesirable. To recognize this point is very important, for it will prevent us from following extreme diets. Every extreme diet results in the loss of nutritional balance, and balance is especially important for fats. Too much of total fat is at the root of several health problems. Eating too much fat over a period of time, especially the saturated fats, can lead to digestion problems and gallbladder disease. Overloading the fat transport mechanism in blood sets the stage for cardiovascular disease.

Furthermore, our fat cells eventually get so stuffed with storage fat that obesity results, which in some individuals can progress to diabetes (the type II type).

But let's face it, fats have also positive sides. They give foods a pleasant taste—some say a good mouth-feel. Fats or oils make bland foods more tasty, help in the absorption of fat-soluble vitamins, and fats give us a happy satisfied feeling after a meal. If we had to store energy in our body in a less condensed form than fat, our body would be huge. To balance the positive and negative sides of our dietary fats, we need to select them wisely and use them in moderation.

The Atherosclerosis Connection

The reason for the mental gymnastics about dietary fat is to a large extent their relationship with atherosclerosis. Atherosclerosis is a disorder of blood vessels in which abnormal fatty streaks are deposited inside the arteries and eventually block blood flow. Although suspected for many years, diet as a causal factor was implicated only during the last few decades. Since the trailblazing studies of Keys and his coworkers (who documented that dietary fat influenced the level of blood cholesterol) and the famous Framingham heart studies (which linked

121

high blood cholesterol to heart attacks), we have learned a great deal about diet and atherosclerosis. One point is clear: fat and cholestrol are main players in the drama and diet must be taken seriously. Innumerable studies have shown that fat-controlled, heart-smart diets are beneficial. We have the knowledge to devise such diets, but for many of us reeducation is necessary. To change firmly entrenched eating habits has been a problem much more difficult than we thought. This reeducation, furthermore, is made difficult because the foods that are most problematic are exactly those that signalled affluence in our culture and have been symbols of the American way of life.

A combination of diet, exercise, and meditation can reverse atherosclerotic lesions.
—A. P. Simopoulos. "Nutrition and Fitness: A Conference Report Nutrition," *Nutrition Today* 27(6) (1992): 24–29.

Cholesterol Is No Fat but Linked to It

In the famous Framingham study begun over forty years ago and still going on, increased risk of heart attacks was related to high blood cholesterol levels. Researchers showed a significant rise in the number of heart attacks when blood cholesterol was higher than 200 mg per 100 ml blood. These and other findings led to the crusade against high blood cholesterol (hyper-cholesterolemia). Today the media—newspapers and TV—tell us that cholesterol is bad for us. Actually cholesterol is a very important and necessary compound in our body. The brain, for exaple, contains a great deal of cholesterol, but because it is so vital for our well-being, our body has the capacity to make all the cholesterol we ever need. Dietary cholesterol in excess only results in overload. So when our blood cholesterol level increases, small amounts of cholesterol and other fatty material get caught on the arterial walls and form atherosclerotic plaque. These deposits can eventually block the blood flow, resulting in a heart attack or a stroke if the blockage is in the brain. Physicians tell us that a high blood cholesterol is a risk factor for atherosclerosis, heart disease, and stroke. The lesson of all this is to keep our blood cholesterol low.

To keep blood cholesterol levels from creeping up to abnormally high levels and reduce the risk for a heart attack and stroke, we must know the factors that keep blood cholesterol in a safe range. As a start, we could exercise—we could walk, jog or swim. Regular moderate exercise lowers blood cholesterol. In addition we also need to review our diets. Would it help to eat differently? Should we improve our diet? This is a more difficult question to answer. We know that diet in part or in whole is responsible for elevated blood cholesterol. But the question is, can we bring down our blood cholesterol level by making appropriate dietary changes?

Less Dietary Cholesterol

If we want to keep our blood cholesterol low, it makes sense to get as little cholesterol as possible from our diets. Egg yolk is by far the major source of cholesterol in American diets. Therefore, decreasing eggs to not more than two per week has been recommended. Besides egg there are a number of other foods that are a potential source of cholesterol. Liver and brain, for example, and to a lesser degree shellfish, are dietary cholesterol sources. However, these foods are usually not eaten frequently. Intermediate sources of dietary cholesterol are meats, chicken, milk, butter. Some foods interfere with the absorption of dietary cholesterol. One such item is the soluble fiber from oatmeal or the pectin from apples and other fruits. This is one of the many reasons to include fiber in our diet. But not all types of fiber seem to have this effect.

Reducing and controlling dietary cholesterol intake is a first step in reducing our blood cholesterol level and therefore in decreasing the risks for atherosclerosis. But alas, the effect of this reduction is less than we would like. Other dietary changes are necessary. To have a significant effect on blood cholesterol reduction, we need to look at the dietary fat in addition to changes in dietary cholesterol.

123

How to Lower Your Blood Cholesterol

The situation with fats is complicated since some types of dietary fats increase and other types of fat decrease blood cholesterol. We do not have a simple explanation why this is so, but innumerable studies have shown that the saturated fats in our diet drive blood cholesterol up, while the polyunsaturated fats drive it down. So if you need to reduce your blood cholesterol, you must reduce the daily intake of saturated fat from beef, pork, lamb, butter, coconut, palm oil, and reduce the fat from chicken and turkey (remove skin), and the partially hydrogenated fats from a variety of margarine and spreads. At the same time, your intake of polyunsaturated fats should increase, partly from vegetable oils and partly from fish. All the while keeping in mind *that the total fat intake should be low.* Just by reducing your total fat and saturated fat intake and including some polyunsaturated fats, you can improve your diet. Such changes will lower blood cholesterol and consequently decrease the risk for atherosclerosis.

Two other risk factors for heart disease and stroke, besides the high blood cholesterol levels, are smoking and high blood pressure. Reducing smoking and controlling your blood pressure, the latter by medication or stress relaxation, are also of great importance in decreasing the risk for heart disease.

Blood Cholesterol—Marker for Heart Disease

Studies in the United States and around the globe have shown that the greater the amount of cholesterol circulating in blood, the greater the chance of a heart attack. Routinely blood-cholesterol levels are checked and diets to decrease blood cholesterol are widely advocated on TV, in newspapers, and on the radio. A ball park figure of 200 mg blood cholesterol/dl is often quoted as a cutoff figure above which diet intervention is started.

However, the situation is not quite that simple. Blood cholesterol slowly increases throughout life and therefore cholesterol standards are needed for different age groups. While a cholesterol of one hundred eighty mg/dl might be acceptable for an older person, the same value in a twenty-year-old would be too high. With further research it also became clear that the cholesterol story was much more complicated than was initially thought. At least two kinds of cholesterol-carrying particles were identified in blood, which sometimes are referred to as the *good* and the *bad* cholesterol. The bad cholesterol ("the low density" or LDL-cholesterol) particles can bind to all kinds of body cells and deposit the cholesterol they carry into cells and unfortunately also onto our artery walls. The good cholesterol ("high density" or HDL-cholesterol) moves the cholesterol from body cells to the liver where it is processed for excretion in bile. Naturally if the HDL removal system works well, we have a more efficient system to get rid of cholesterol and this will keep our blood cholesterol low and therefore also lower the risk of heart attacks and strokes. Men are usually more prone to heart attacks because their removal system seems less efficient than that of women who have more of the beneficial HDL than men. After menopause, women lose this protection and their risk for heart disease is similar to that for men. Exercise improves the effectiveness of cholesterol disposal (HDL) in both men and women.

Table 14

Guidelines for Blood Cholesterol Levels

Type of Cholesterol	Desirable	High Risk for CHD*
Total cholesterol (mg/dl)	Less than 200	More than 240
LDL (bad) cholesterol (mg/dl)	Less than 130	More than 130
HDL (good) cholesterol (mg/dl)	More than 60	Less than 35

*Cholesterol levels that indicate high risk for coronary heart disease.

—E. J. Schaefer, M.D., *Nutrition Review* (1993) 51: 246–252.

However, blood cholesterol testing may not tell the whole story for everybody. According to Dr. Castelli, noted physician of the Framingham Heart Study, some individuals who have low cholesterol but high fat levels (triglycerides) in their blood may also be at risk for heart disease. That other factors besides cholesterol are involved in reducing the risks for a heart attack is also shown by the effects of fish oils, which not only affect blood cholesterol but also have a beneficial effect on blood clotting. All these findings tell us that atherosclerosis is a complex disorder. They further highlight the importance of diet, especially our fat intake, in relationship to chronic disease.

The National Cholesterol Education Program Expert Panel on Cholesterol in Children Recommends Cholesterol Screening for:
**Offspring of parents and grandparents who suffered before 55 years of age premature atherosclerosis, a heart attack, angina pectoris, peripheral vascular disease, or sudden death.
**Offspring of parents who have blood cholesterol higher than 240 mg/dl.
**Children whose parental medical history is unobtainable.
    —L. Snetselaar Laur RM. "Childhood, Diet and the Atherosclerotic Process," *Nutrition Today* 27 (1) (1992): 22–28

Dietary Fat Makes a Difference

The recognition that diet and lifestyle are important not only in the prevention of heart disease but in several other diseases of civilization has led to a revolution in our dietary practices. We have made many changes, but we still have some way to go and perhaps we will never come to the point where we get maximum benefit from dietary protection. Those who have made changes toward a more healthy lifestyle tell of very positive effects on their well-being, stamina, and health. While the changes cannot guarantee the prevention of *all disease*, they may go a long way to decrease the risk for chronic disease and to improve the quality of and outlook on life.

The dietary guidelines put forth by the nutrition, medical, and scientific community suggest limiting total and saturated fat in our diet. The three groups of foods that need to be particularly scrutinized are the meat group, the dairy group, and the many foods that contain hidden sources of fat. If you plan your diet according to the guidelines and obtain the recommended portions from the food guide, you already know you need to trim fat from meats, and to select low-fat dairy products. To control fat from these two food groups will affect and decrease your saturated fat. If you add any fat during cooking, use olive oil, always sparingly, and a polyunsaturated oil as salad dressing. The new food labels with information on total and saturated fat content will help us to find the "hidden fat" in foods.

Before you start label reading for fat, saturated fats, and cholesterol, find out how much fat is about right for you. Caloric requirements vary from person to person, and this influences the amount of dietary fat. Therefore diets must be tailor-made to your individual needs. In figure 10 the upper limits of daily total fat and saturated fat intakes are given for three diets at different calorie levels. An obese person eating the recommended servings who wants to limit calories to, say 1,400 Cal per day, should get less than fifty g total fat and less than 15 saturated fat per day. On the other hand, an extremely active person with a high energy requirement of 2,600 Cal should get less than 85 g total, of which less than 30 g should be saturated fat. For healthy, average, moderately active persons, requiring approximately 2,000 Cal per day, the limit would be 65 g of total fat and 20 g of saturated fat per day.

Labels Worth Reading

The new FDA regulations on food labels place the nutrients that are of greatest *Public Health* significance first. Of the fourteen mandatory nutrients, the first five relate to fat and cholesterol: they are calories, calories from fat, grams total fat, grams

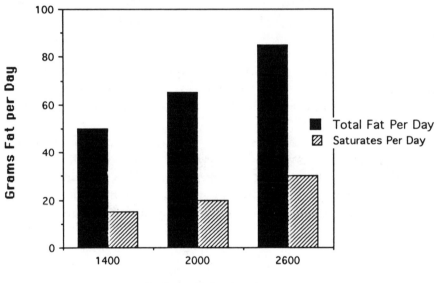

Keep Your Fat and Saturates Below these Levels

Figure 10

A

Nutrition Facts
Serving Size ½ cup (114g)
Servings Per Container 4

Amount Per Serving

Calories 90   Calories from Fat 30

	% Daily Value*
Total Fat 3g	**5%**
Saturated Fat 0g	**0%**
Cholesterol 0mg	**0%**
Sodium 300mg	**13%**
Total Carbohydrate 13g	**4%**
Dietary Fiber 3g	**12%**
Sugars 3g	
Protein 3g	

Vitamin A	80%	•	Vitamin C	60%
Calcium	4%	•	Iron	4%

* Percent Daily Values are based on a 2,000 calorie diet. Your daily values may be higher or lower depending on your calorie needs:

		Calories	2,000	2,500
Total Fat	Less than		65g	80g
Sat Fat	Less than		20g	25g
Cholesterol	Less than		300mg	300mg
Sodium	Less than		2,400mg	2,400mg
Total Carbohydrate			300g	375g
Fiber			25g	30g

Calories per gram:
Fat 9   •   Carbohydrate 4   •   Protein 4

B

Serving Size 1 cup (228g)
Servings Per Container 2

Amount Per Serving

Calories 260   Calories from Fat 120

	% Daily Value*
Total Fat 13g	**20%**
Saturated Fat 5g	**25%**
Cholesterol 30mg	**10%**
Sodium 660mg	**28%**
Total Carbohydrate 31g	**10%**
Dietary Fiber 0g	**0%**
Sugars 5g	
Protein 5g	

Vitamin A 4%	•	Vitamin C 2%
Calcium 15%	•	Iron 4%

* Percent Daily Values are based on a 2,000 calorie diet. Your daily values may be higher or lower depending on your calorie needs:

		Calories:	2,000	2,500
Total Fat	Less than		65g	80g
Sat Fat	Less than		20g	25g
Cholesterol	Less than		300mg	300mg
Sodium	Less than		2,400mg	2,400mg
Total Carbohydrate			300g	375g
Dietary Fiber			25g	30g

Calories per gram:
Fat 9 • Carbohydrate 4 • Protein 4

C

Nutrition Facts
Serving Size 1 can (360 mL)

Amount Per Serving

Calories 140

	% Daily Value*
Total Fat 0g	**0%**
Sodium 20mg	**1%**
Total Carbohydrate 36g	**12%**
Sugars 36 g	
Protein 0g	**0%**

* Percent Daily Values are based on a 2,000 calorie diet.

Figure 11 *

*Danielle Shor and Charles Edwards, "USDA's Role: Nutrition Labeling of Meat and Poultry Products," *Nutrition Today* 28 (5) 1993: 25 (reprinted by permission).

saturated fat, and mg cholesterol. In addition to the mandatory information on total fat, manufacturers may voluntarily state the calories from polyunsaturated fats and monounsaturated fats (see figure 11).

To use the food label information about fats to good advantage, first look at the serving size of figure11. In our example of labels A, B, and C, the respective serving sizes are half a cup, one cup, and one can. If you eat more than one serving, you need to adjust all other nutrition information (for two servings, double the amount of fat, for example). Calories are given per serving as well as the calories coming from fat. Product A provides 30 Cal from fat, B provides 120, and C is a fat-free product, since all the calories come from sugar. Total fat is listed in grams and as a percentage of the recommended limit of a 2,000 Cal-a-day diet. If per serving the "percent daily value" is less than 5 percent, the food is considered a low-fat food. Look also for a low-percent daily value for saturated fat as well as for cholesterol and sodium. Remember that the percentages of daily values have been computed for a 2,000-Cal diet. For lower calorie diets, adjust downward; for higher calorie diets, you may slightly increase the fat.

The new labels give a great deal of helpful nutrition information about food products to the consumer. When you first read labels about fat, it may be somewhat cumbersome. By way of introduction, concentrate on the grams of fat, the grams of saturated fats, and the amount of cholesterol in a product. Looking at these items on the labels in Figure 11, you see immediately that product B is high in fat. Furthermore, product A does not contain any saturated fat, while B is a significant source of saturated fat and cholesterol. The ingredient list of a food will give further information on the origin of fat (such as soy, tropical seeds, coconut, lard, etc.) which together with the mandated food label will give a wealth of useful nutrition information to plan healthful diets.

Food Descriptors You Will Find on Food Labels

A *LOW FAT* food has three grams or less of fat per serving.

A *Low Saturated Fat* food has less than one gram of saturated fat per serving.

A *Low-Calorie* food provides forty calories or less.

Light means a food item has only one-third the calories or the fat of its conventional counterpart.

Reduced means a food has 25 percent fewer calories, fat, or sodium than the regular product.

Free means a food provides less than one-half gram of fat per serving or an insignificant amount.

Step Nine: Fat Affects More than Your Heart

The area we need to be most concerned about relates to our dietary fat. Fats have of course their place in every diet, but they need to be watched. If you have read the previous chapters and are choosing your food in line with the food group recommendations, you are already on the right track since all along we have stressed the selection of low-fat items. What remains is to make sure to choose the right type of fat.

To get started review briefly how many calories your diet should approximately provide. This is important because fat intake is related to the total calories you need. If you are a person of small stature, fairly inactive, or obese, a low-calorie diet is appropriate. With increasing body size and increasing activity, a person will require more calories and consequently fat intake can be more liberal. Remember a 2,000-Cal diet has been taken as reference on all food labels, which is a diet for a moderately active nonobese person. You need either to decrease or increase depending on your own situation. For a low-calorie diet of approximately 1,400 Cal per day, the total fat should be less than 45 g and saturated fat less than 15 g per day. High-calorie diets providing food for extremely active people can have somewhat more total and saturated fat.

Now that you have determined the maximum total and saturated fat level that is appropriate for you, food-label reading becomes a must at least until you are used to a healthful selection of foods. As you go through the day, write down on a paper the type of food you have eaten, the serving size of the food, and the grams of total fat and of saturated fat in the serving. At the end of the day, total the amounts for total and saturated fat. Both should be below the limit you have worked out. If your fat intake is above your limit, try again the next day and shoot for a little less fat the following day. Very soon you will learn which foods to choose, which foods to eat less frequently, or which low-fat items you can substitute for those of high saturated fat content.

The next point is to make sure to include sufficient polys and monos. Since the polys can be damaged by heat exposure, their use as cooking oils should be minimized. Olive oil with a preponderance of monos is somewhat more resistant to heat, and if you have recipes that call for cooking fat, you can use this oil sparingly for food preparation. The polyunsaturated fats, such as safflower, canola, sunflower, soybean, and corn oil are best used in salads and in recipes that do not expose fat to high heat. Vegetables, for example, can be steamed briefly in little water and the oil added after cooking for taste and better absorption of fat-soluble vitamins. Never smother any food with oil. When you pour oil from a bottle, use a spoon to measure the desired quantity.

To obtain the omega-3 fats from ocean fish, include one or two three-ounce portions of fish per week to provide these fats. Soybean and canola oil also provide a small amount of the omega-3 fats. Using these for salads is a good idea. Since the fish oils are damaged by heat, cook fish briefly by steaming or in a nonstick pan with the least addition of fat.

Any extreme in the selection of fat may well lead to problems. Very low fat diets have been suggested for the therapy of atherosclerosis. Diets like the Pritikin diet are very low in fat, difficult to prepare, and may not be very palatable when first introduced. Extremely low fat diets may not provide enough of the essential fatty acids from polys, which are required by the body. With reeducation under the direction of a dietitian as to how to prepare them, such diets can benefit some individuals. For everyday use and for the great majority of individuals in the United States, such drastic measures are not called for. However, some modification of the fat in our diets is extremely desirable. To use the many fats and oils intelligently and to minimize detrimental effects on health, four points need to be stressed:

1. Select lean or low fat items from **the meat and dairy** group. This will reduce your total as well as your saturated dietary fat.
2. For salads, select oils that provide the polys.
3. If you use an oil for cooking, use olive oil with least heat exposure. The polys are affected by heat.
4. Obtain some of the omega-3 fats from fish and from soybean or canola oils.

Lastly a word about dietary cholesterol. In theory we do not need any in our diet because it is not an essential nutrient. But since cholesterol is part of foods in our diet, it is recommended that we limit their major source to two eggs per week.

For You to Do

1. Start reading food labels to get used to information about fat.

2. Find out how much fat and saturated fat your diet provides.

3. Is your fat intake in line with the recommendation?

4. If you need to reduce your total and saturated fat, what foods could you substitute? Write down the foods that are most problematic in your diet.

5. Make a long-term plan to eat in line with the recommendations.

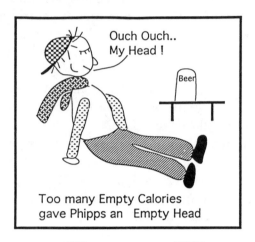

Chapter XI
Alcohol—
Source of Empty Calories

Besides fat, carbohydrates, and protein, the only other source of calories in our diet is alcohol. However, alcohol is not really a food. It provides empty calories, is a drug because of its depressing effect on the brain, and is a teratogen because it can induce birth defects in the offspring of pregnant women who consume alcohol during critical periods of fetal development, especially in the first trimester.

Alcohol differs significantly from the other energy nutrients since it has powerful and detrimental effects on the human body. Alcohol often displaces other nutrient-dense foods in the diet that provide vitamins and minerals. Too much alcohol interferes with the absorption of nutrients from the diet and has multiple effects on human organs and tissues. The liver is the only organ that can break down ingested alcohol and long-term excessive alcohol consumption results in irreversible damage to liver cells and impaired liver function.

Weight for weight pure alcohol provides more calories than carbohydrates, but fewer than fat (7-Cal g alcohol). If alcohol calories displace foods and supply a significant portion of the day's caloric intake, too many empty calories are ingested. A varied, balanced, and adequate diet with moderate alcohol consumption has minimal detrimental effects on health. Excessive consumption of alcohol, in addition to the depressing effects on the brain, almost always interferes with nutrients and leads eventually to deficiencies of vitamins and minerals.

As a quick reference for the caloric content of common alcoholic beverages, the amount of alcohol in beer is 4 to 6 percent, of wine 9 to 12 percent, and distilled eighty-proof liquor is approximately 40 percent pure alcohol. This would mean an 8-ounce can of beer will provide 99 Cal, a 3-ounce glass of wine 63 Cal, and one shot of liquor (1.5 ounce) 126 alcohol Cal. Alcohol calories are considered empty calories (see table 15).

Table 15
Calorie Content of Alcoholic Beverages

Type of Beverage	Fluid oz	Calories
Beer	8.0	99
Beer	12.0	148
Ale	8.0	98
Wine, dessert, dry, 18.8%	3.5	126
Wine, dessert, sweet, 18.8%	3.5	153
Sauterne, California	3.5	84
Table wine, red, 11.5%	3.5	76
Table wine, white, 11.5%	3.5	80
Champagne dry	4.0	84
Champagne sweet	4.0	160
Sherry	2.0	84
Vermouth, dry	3.5	105
Cordials	1.0	97
Gin, rum, vodka, whisky		
80 proof	1.0	65
100 proof	1.0	83
Gin rickey	4.0	150
Manhattan	3.5	164
Martini	3.5	140
Whisky sour	2.5	138

Step Ten: If You Use Alcohol . . .

To those who like alcoholic beverages, moderation must be the overriding concern. Any excessive use of alcohol not only will lead to long-term severe health problems but also to all kinds of short-term problems, such as hangovers, accidents, lost time, interpersonal problems, and loss of human dignity. Using table 15 (see page 136), compute the alcohol calories you have consumed per day. If alcohol provides more than 200 Cal per day, you receive a significant portion of your daily calories from alcohol. Too many empty calories and too much interference by alcohol with your normal nutritional processes lead to dietary deficiencies. Alcohol, for example, acts as a diuretic, enhancing the elimination of water-soluble nutrients.

If you drink, drink an alcoholic beverage at mealtime. The depressing effect on the body is somewhat blunted by the food. If you cannot stop drinking, better never start. If you have a problem with alcohol, recognize it and seek help. Early intervention can prevent the irreversible damage to the liver and the multiple nutritional deficiencies that result from chronic alcoholism. As with nutrients, moderation and balance are the keys in the use of alcohol.

How to Be a Good Host and Hostess

Offer soft drinks. One-third of the adult population chooses not to drink at all.

Give more than a drink. Introduce people to each other, get conversation going. You have more to give than just drinks.

Don't rush refills. Wait until glass is empty before offering more.

Don't double up. A lot of people count their drinks. If you double, they drink twice as much.

Dinner is served. Serve dinner before it is too late. If cocktail hour goes on and on nobody will remember what was served for dinner.

Keep them nibbling. Not just later on but while guests are drinking. It slows down the rate at which people drink.

If someone drinks too much, you are responsible. Keep the guest in your home or make arrangements to get them home safely. Only time can sober him/her up.

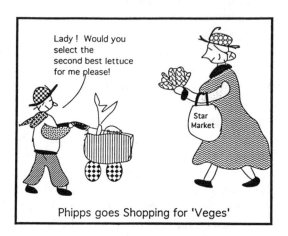

Phipps goes Shopping for 'Veges'

Chapter XII
Vitamins for Good Health

Only a few years back, many families had a vitamin bottle on the breakfast table and adults and children took a vitamin pill as a matter of course on a daily basis. This practice was based on the erroneous assumption that a vitamin pill a day would enable us to be well nourished. Today we know better. Vitamin pills have some benefits for some people, but they will not guarantee that our nutritional needs are met.

So if pills are not the answer, how can we be sure to receive all our daily vitamins? As we shall see in this section, a good diet can provide all the vitamins we require. The preoccupation with vitamins by professionals and the public alike during the first part of this century came about because of the spectacular discoveries of vitamin deficiency conditions and how to prevent them. For centuries humankind had been plagued by devastating vitamin deficiencies. Only sixty years ago, pellagra—the dietary deficiency of the B vitamin niacin—was responsible for many patients in New York's mental institutions. Pellagra was called the "Four D's" (dermatitis, diarrhea, dementia, and death) and in painstaking studies was shown to be the result of a deficiency of the B vitamin niacin. The discovery that a single vitamin cured and prevented such a devastating condition subconsciously gave faith in vitamins.

Vitamins Are Big Business

---

40 percent of Americans supplement their diets, resulting in $3.5 billion annual sales or $9.5 million each day.

Historical documents show that people in practically every country have experienced at one time or other similar tragedies related to one or several nutrients. In Britain and in other countries, children suffered from rickets, a vitamin-deficiency condition now preventable by vitamin D. Entire Swiss village populations were deficient in iodine and were doomed to live their lives with goiter and some, as cretins. Fortification of salt with iodine prevented this disorder in Switzerland and in many other countries. The disease of rice-eating countries in the Far East was beriberi, a nervous disorder claiming many lives. Beriberi was caused by a vitamin B_1 deficiency in people living on polished rice. It was cured and prevented simply by switching from polished to whole-grain rice, which provided the vitamin. Many more examples could be cited, such as the fascinating story of scurvy, the disease of sailors caused by a vitamin C deficiency, which occurred during long sea voyages. In all these instances, improved vitamin or mineral nutrition made the difference between sickness and health. It was not surprising that such spectacular feats had assured vitamin pills a prominent place on our breakfast tables!

But should we use vitamins from a bottle? After all they are cheap and we can get them in fairly concentrated form as "insurance" to prevent deficiency. For one, if we rely on vitamin pills, we get complacent and erroneously assume that our diets are adequate. Another reason against the indiscriminate use of concentrated vitamin preparations is their potential toxicity. Any vitamin consumed in large quantities is a potential poison. The toxicity of long-term excesses of vitamin A and D has been well documented. Even the water-soluble vitamins, which we thought to be fairly nontoxic, in high amounts can produce serious health hazards when high-potency pills are taken over some period of time. The confusing number of vitamin pills on the market also vary in their vitamin composition and may lack one or several vitamins that are essential while others are provided in excessive amounts. Most importantly, though, is that our diets must provide vitamins together with other nutrients in a natural balance. Such a balance is obtained from wholesome unrefined foods and may be lost if we get our vitamins from pills.

Supplementing the diet is generally a personal decision for those who believe they do not get all of the nutrients they need from the diet.
—V. Srinivasan, et al. *Nutrition Today* **28(6)** (1993): 28–33.

Vitamins Alone Can't Do the Job

In the United States today everybody is familiar with vitamins and they need no introduction. Less known is why we need them and what their function is in our body. In a nutshell vitamins are catalysts that carry out many complicated reactions. To define their function in one single sentence over and above their catalytic role is impossible because each of the vitamins has unique, usually many, and most intricate functions. Several B vitamins, for example, are required in the liberation of energy from foods, but the vitamins themselves do not provide energy. Our body machinery is like a complicated clockwork; vitamins must be present in proper concentration at the right time so that it can work. Just consider for a minute the synthesis of the hormone insulin or the immune globulins. If we want to make insulin in pancreatic cells or the immune globulins in specific white blood cells, we need the amino acids as building blocks, we also need the energy from carbohydrates to fuel the protein synthesis machinery, and we need vitamins to direct and facilitate the complicated processes involved. Should either the building blocks, the energy, or the vitamins be in short supply, our body machinery does not run smoothly. This is similar to building a house—which requires building material, labor to build, and a supervisor to direct the operations. Whole, healthful diets provide all the body requires. Wholesome food provides vitamins, minerals, protein, and energy from carbohydrate and fat in good balance so that body processes can progress with the efficient use of all food components.

Vitamins from Food

If our diet is varied and limits empty calories, we have come a long way in obtaining our vitamins. Each of the five food groups is a significant source of one or several vitamins. Whole grains, bread and cereals, as well as items made from fortified flour are good sources of several B vitamins. The fruit and vegetable groups are excellent sources of vitamin C, folate, vitamin B_1, and vitamin

K. Foods from the dairy group are good sources of vitamin D, A, and riboflavin, and all animal foods provide vitamin B_6 and B_{12} and contribute greatly to our dietary niacin requirement.

Eating from the Food Groups Is Good for Your Vitamins

Whole grains provide vitamin B_1
Fruits and vegetables provide vitamins C, K,
    beta-carotene, and folacin
Milk provides vitamin A, D, and riboflavin
Meats provide niacin, vitamin B_6, and B_{12}
Vegetable oils provide vitamin E

To eat from the food groups according to the guidelines results in diets that are surprisingly well balanced in terms of vitamins. Such diets certainly will prevent vitamin deficiencies and in most cases even provide "luxury" amounts of vitamins. Vitamins obtained from diets rather than from pills also prevent excessive intakes and potential vitamin toxicities. Such diets are safe, sound, and aid our well-being. They give satisfaction through their taste and curb excessive hunger.

Two or three points are absolutely vital to remember. At least twice a week, eat a serving of *dark green leafy vegetables.* They provide folic acid, which is sometimes a problem in U.S. diets. Every day eat a serving of *green leafy and / or yellow vegetables.* This will provide beta-carotene, a precursor of vitamin A, which has antioxidant properties independent of vitamin A. Researchers think that by some unknown mechanism the antioxidants—vitamin A, beta-carotene, and other carotenoids, vitamin E, and vitamin C—aid in the prevention of some cancers (and possibly a long list of other diseases still not well studied).

A daily good source of *vitamin C* is also a must, such as a serving of citrus fruit or juice. Be sure to buy pure juice. Orange drinks to which vitamin C is added do not contain other nutrients, such as potassium or soluble fiber. Some vegetables are also excellent sources of vitamin C. A serving of broccoli or of green pepper, for example, has the equivalent vitamin C of an orange, provided the vegetable is not overcooked.

Choosing the recommended servings from the food groups. Make sure you get every day:

1. A serving of a vitamin C-rich fruit or vegetable
2. A serving of yellow or green vegetables and
3. A serving of dark green vegetables twice a week.

Vitamins are delicate substances. Storing and cooking can damage them. Water-soluble vitamins leach out into cooking water and are thus lost. Vitamin B_6, riboflavin, and vitamin K are damaged by light. Therefore, storage and cooking methods are critical to the vitamin content of foods.

To get the most from the vitamins in foods, keep in mind to:

· store vegetables in the refrigerator

· cook vegetables with the least amount of water, preferably steam vegetables

· not add baking soda to green vegetables to retain their green color. The alkalinity of baking soda will destroy vitamin C and vitamin B_1.

· cook vegetables the shortest time possible (broccoli cooked eight minutes is just right and 80 percent of vitamin C is retained. Cooking for twenty minutes destroys 80 percent of the vitamin C in broccoli).

· serve vegetables immediately.

Are You at Risk?

For centuries people have survived on diets without the use of vitamin pills, proving that diet alone can provide all the vitamins we need. On the other hand, all through history some populations have suffered from vitamin deficiency diseases and there are children in Asian and Central American populations who even today become blind because they are deficient in vitamin A. We have today an almost astronomical armament of vitamin preparations, confusing combinations of vitamins with different potencies, some combined with minerals and nonnutrient substances. The question is who needs these preparations and which one is the best?

Before we can answer such a question, we need to look at our diet. Our first concern should be to ask whether our diet is adequate. If we eat junk food or follow odd diets that eliminate whole food groups, a vitamin pill may help some, but will not be the whole answer. In fact such supplements give us a false security if we assume that they rectify bad food habits. Before we take vitamin pills, we need to look critically at our total diet. Without improving diets in variety, balance, moderation, and controlling for fat, sugar, and salt, vitamin pills do very little for us. We need a balance of calorie-providing foods, protein, fiber, vitamins, minerals, and sufficient fluid in our diet.

With the development of many modern food products, traditional diets have been changing rapidly. New foods have been engineered, the ever-increasing abundance of supermarket foods provides us with a year round supply of a great variety of foods. Most people who plan adequate diets have no need for vitamin pills, but there are exceptions. The U.S. population groups that might benefit from vitamin pills because they are at risk for problems related to vitamins are the following:

1. People who are dieting and cutting down their calories to fewer than 1,200 Cal per day. Even if they select foods of high-nutrient density, those people will not be able to satisfy their daily need for vitamins and minerals. During such periods of dieting, a supplement of

144

all vitamins and minerals in concentrations of 100 percent of the RDA is helpful.

2. Another group are the elderly. During aging the energy requirement decreases while the requirement for many nutrients, including vitamins, may increase. Although many elderly are consuming adequate diets, others do not adapt to these changing requirements. Elderly persons who are not motivated, have difficulties in adjusting to living alone, have limited finances, or may need medications that interfere with nutrients, may not consume adequate diets. Some, but by no means all, elderly as a group are at greater risk for vitamin deficiencies and/or other nutritional inadequacies. A vitamin supplement may help in part, but adjustment of the whole diet is necessary.

3. People who eat diets high in refined foods are also candidates for vitamin problems. Refining of grains results in loss of their native micronutrient and fiber content. The use of excess sugar, which is a highly refined product providing empty calories, may induce vitamin deficiencies as well as excessive loss from the body of some trace mineral elements. A vitamin/mineral supplement can give an initial boost, but a change to more wholesome, high density foods is absolutely necessary to get long-term health benefits.

4. Consuming excess alcohol, too, interferes with the nutrition of a person. Total food intake may decrease in alcoholics. Alcohol interferes with nutrient absorption from the gut. Alcohol is also a diuretic and will increase the loss of water-soluble vitamins, magnesium, and zinc among other nutrients in urine. Vitamin supplements can be helpful, but again a vitamin pill *alone* will not be the answer. A healthful total diet, reduced alcohol intake, together with a vitamin/mineral supplement is the answer.

5. People who are sick often have special nutritional requirements and individuals with gastrointestinal problems are specifically at risk for nutrient absorption problems. Ask the physician what supplements would be helpful. During recuperation a one-a-day type supplement of vitamins and minerals may be suggested by the physician.

6. Individuals who are on long-term medications that interfere with one or several nutrients. Drug-nutrient interactions are common and need to be addressed by the attending physician.

Synthetic versus Natural Vitamins

People often distinguish between natural and synthetic vitamins. Be sure to get the natural one, the one from rose hips and not the chemical, made in a test tube! In most cases this is a fallacy. Vitamin C made in the chemist's test tube is exactly the same as the vitamin C in rose hips. Some synthetic vitamins may be even somewhat superior to the ones from food. Folic acid from a vitamin pill is in the free form and is well absorbed by our gut while the bound form from foods is sometimes less well absorbed. On the other hand, some vitamins such as vitamin E may differ depending whether the vitamin comes from a pill or from food, since there are many different forms of the vitamin in nature. In general, however, the distinction of synthetic and natural is not useful. All vitamins are chemicals and the argument against synthetic vitamins—that they are chemicals—is not appropriate. The problem with some of the natural vitamin preparations is that their amounts are not well defined. Sometimes the concentrations of vitamins in these products are very high and may result in toxicities in susceptible individuals, such as vitamin D from cod liver oil.

Many elders suffer from nutritional excesses and/or toxicities from vitamin and mineral supplement overuse.
—J. Dwyer, "Strategies to Detect and Prevent Malnutrition in the Elderly,"
Nutrition Today 29(5) (1994): 14–24.

Many examples demonstrating the complexity of vitamin nutrition could be cited. Without a thorough study of vitamins, many of our ideas about them are clichés, which on greater inspection do not hold up. What is applicable to one vitamin is erroneous for another, for each vitamin has unique functions and one cannot substitute for another. Some vitamins are stored in our liver, such as the fat-soluble vitamins A, D, E, and K, while the water-soluble vitamins are easily lost in urine. The fat-soluble vitamins ingested in too high amounts can produce variable toxicities and disease. Excess water-soluble vitamins also can be toxic, but less so, since they are more easily excreted.

Selecting a Vitamin Supplement

If you are in the group of individuals at risk for vitamin problems, you might want to take a vitamin supplement. But which one? Are there guidelines to select the best, safest, and cheapest preparation?

First check what's in the preparation. If you think you need a vitamin supplement because you are dieting or you feel run down, select a preparation that provides all the vitamins and minerals as 100 percent of the Recommended Dietary Allowances (U.S. RDAs). Together with your diet the amount equal to 100 percent of recommendations is ample and there is little chance of getting toxic amounts as long as you take only one pill per day.

Label reading is especially important when you buy a vitamin preparation. Some types have very odd vitamin compositions, which do not make sense (some vitamins excessively high and other missing). Unless there is a medical reason for such a preparation, stay away from preparations that provide more than the RDA, sometimes as high as ten times the amount recommended. Any vitamin prescribed as a medical treatment needs to be taken as prescribed. For example, the long-term indiscriminate use of high vitamin A preparations for acne has resulted in severe toxicities, such as continuous severe headaches in individuals who took this preparation unsupervised for extended periods.

Experience has shown that people who need a vitamin supplement also need essential trace elements. Therefore vitamin/mineral supplements should provide amounts equal to 100 percent of the U.S. RDA, or the usual, safe intake for those trace elements for which no RDA has been determined.

Step Eleven: Get All the Vitamins You Need

First, go back to our diet sample of 1,612 Cal (table 7) and evaluate the contribution of vitamins to this one-day intake. The data show very clearly that a diet selected according to the food guide even on the lowest calorie diet will provide sufficient vitamins if compared to the adult RDAs. Vitamins A and C are present in even higher than RDA requirements. Of course, vitamin intakes will vary from day to day, but such variations are to be expected and reflect the variety of foods chosen on consecutive days.

Since most diets provide more calories than the 1,612-Cal sample, it stands to reason that if you increase the number of portions from the grain and vegetable group, you would increase some of your vitamins and minerals also. With increasing calories and selecting foods from the food groups rather than empty calorie items, more than sufficient vitamins are obtained.

Even if we select some food items that provide some empty calories in addition to this diet, the vitamins still would be adequate. However, there is a limit to the inclusion of empty calories. Eventually we will have less and less vitamins available and our diet gets progressively out of balance. Keep the following five simple criteria in mind when you evaluate your vitamin adequacy:

* Contents of a Vitamin/Mineral Supplement
Note:
The vitamins are present as 100 % of the RDA

EACH TABLET CONTAINS: For Adults– Percentage of U.S. Recommended Daily Allowance (U.S. RDA)

VITAMINS	U.S. RDA		MINERALS		U.S. RDA	MINERALS(con't.)	
Vitamin A			Calcium	162 mg	(16%)	Chloride	36.3 mg*
(as Acetate and			Phosphorus	109 mg	(11%)	Chromium	25 mcg*
Beta Carotene)	5000 IU	(100%)	Iodine	150 mcg	(100%)	Molybdenum	25 mcg*
Vitamin D	400 IU	(100%)	Iron	18 mg	(100%)	Selenium	20 mcg*
Vitamin E	30 IU	(100%)	Magnesium	100 mg	(25%)	Nickel	5 mcg*
Vitamin K₁	25 mcg*		Copper	2 mg	(100%)	Tin	10 mcg*
Vitamin C	60 mg	(100%)	Zinc	15 mg	(100%)	Silicon	2 mg*
Folic Acid	400 mcg	(100%)	Manganese	2.5 mg*		Vanadium	10 mcg*
Vitamin B₁	1.5 mg	(100%)	Potassium	40 mg*		Boron	150 mcg*
Vitamin B₂	1.7 mg	(100%)					
Niacinamide	20 mg	(100%)				*No U.S. RDA established.	
Vitamin B₆	2 mg	(100%)					
Vitamin B₁₂	6 mcg	(100%)					
Pantothenic Acid	10 mg	(100%)					
Biotin	30 mcg	(10 %)					

Inactive Ingredients FD&C Yellow No 6, Hydroxypropyl Methylcellulose,
Lactose, Magnesium Stearate, Microcrystalline Cellulose, Polysorbate 80,
Polyvinylpyrrolidone, Stearic Acid, Titanium Dioxide and Triethyl Citrate.

Figure 12

*Reprinted with permission from RECOMMENDED DIETARY ALLOW-
ANCES: 10TH EDITION. Copyright 1989 by the National Academy of Sciences. Courtesy of the National Academy Press, Washington, D.C.

1. Select the recommended servings from each food group as outlined in previous chapters. Vary the food selected from each food group from day to day.

2. Keep items from the "empty calories" to a minimum. Use sugar only for flavoring. Since oil is rich in polyunsaturated fats, some should be included on a daily basis.

3. Prepare vegetables and fruits to retain their vitamins. Use fresh or frozen produce. Steam vegetables or cook in little water. Do not overcook. Use timer for vegetable cooking. Follow cooking instructions for frozen vegetables.

4. Use yellow and dark green vegetables frequently, preferably every day, for folate, vitamin K, and beta-carotene. Include green leafy vegetables at least twice per week.

5. Make sure you include a good source of vitamin C daily.

Specifics for You to Do

First, as an exercise, check how our 1,612-Cal sample diet (table 7) compares to the five points above:

Our diet includes all recommended servings; criterion 1 is satisfied.

Our diet uses no items from the empty calorie group except low-Cal dressing, olive oil, and butter. Criterion 2 is satisfactory.

We do not know how the food was prepared, so we cannot be sure about point 3. However, the fruit and a salad required no cooking. Therefore we can assume that 3 is satisfactory.

Our diet has two yellow/red vegetables, one green vegetable, and a wedge of lettuce. 4 is satisfactory, except that there is no dark green leafy vegetable included. It is not necessary to eat a dark green leafy vegetable every day. Twice a week would be adequate.

Our diet has at least two good sources of vitamin C, orange juice and broccoli, so 5 is amply satisfied.

How Does Your Own Diet Compare?

Check your own diet and evaluate whether your own vitamin needs are met. In relation to questions 1 through 5, look at your own food intake to see how it compares. If you find that you are missing one or several points, improve your diet in future. The following will guide you:

6. Do you get the reocmmended servings from the food groups?
   Yes ———— Good for you.
   No ———— Go back to better diet planning.

7. Have you selected many foods high in fat and sugar, and alcoholic beverages?
   Yes ———— Go back and review food groups for better food selection.
   No ———— Good for you.

8. Have you received at least three vegetable and two fruit servings per day?
   Yes ———— Good for you.
   No ———— Include more of these groups, some fresh, vegetables not over-cooked.

9. Have you eaten at least one dark green vegetable within the last three days?
   Yes ———— Good for you.
   No ———— Include more of these.

10. Does your diet include a daily source of vitamin C?
    Yes ———— Good for you.
    No ———— Good sources of vitamin C are all citrus fruits and juices, green pepper, broccoli among many other sources.

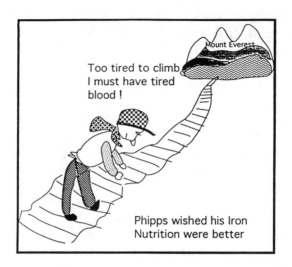

Chapter XIII
Balancing Mineral Nutrients

Our diet must provide as many as twenty different mineral nutrients. Only by eating a variety of foods, as suggested by the food guide, are we likely to obtain all these essential nutrients.

Mineral nutrients, as the vitamins, are needed in comparatively small amounts and do not provide us with energy. Almost all have multiple functions in our body. Calcium and phosphorus are part of bone structure. Iron is necessary to form the hemoglobin in red blood cells. Other mineral nutrients act as catalysts for innumerable vital body reactions. And yet others have regulatory functions, such as sodium in regulating body fluids. From these few examples, we see that the mineral nutrients have varied and unique functions, which are vital to our well-being.

Our diet must provide the mineral nutrients in optimum amounts. Intakes too low or too high produce imbalances, which in either case result in disease. A large number of the mineral nutrients—the trace elements—are required by the body in extremely small daily quantities of only a few milligrams (the size of a pinhead) or less. Toxicities from even small excesses can occur during self-medication with supplements. Another reason to prevent imbalances that might occur by supplementation is that an excess of one mineral nutrient can interfere with the proper function of another. Too much zinc, for example, produces a copper deficiency. The resultant copper deficiency in turn leads to low iron levels in blood, a cause for anemia. Mineral interrelationships of this type are common, and we are only just beginning to understand them. Practically any of the trace elements in excess can become toxic. However, as long as we select a variety of the proposed servings from the grain, vegetable, fruit, dairy, and meat groups, such imbalances are probably unlikely. Wholesome food provides these mineral nutrients in balance without the likelihood of either extreme deficiency or toxicity.

All Five Food Groups Provide Mineral Nutrients

Vegetables and fruits
  Good for trace elements, magnesium, potassium
Whole grains and cereals
  Good for selenium and many other trace elements
Meat group
  Red meats good for iron and zinc
  Seafood for iodine
  Beans for magnesium
Dairy group
  Excellent for calcium and phosphorus
  Good for zinc

Our knowledge of many aspects of mineral nutrition is still fragmentary, yet powerful arguments can be made for several of these nutrients in relation to chronic disease. Among these are sodium and hypertension, calcium and osteoporosis, iron and anemia, fluoride and tooth decay, iodine and goiter, or zinc in delayed wound healing and tissue repair in the elderly. The question is how can we be sure that our mineral nutrition is adequate to decrease the risks for such disorders? Let's consider what we need to do to make sure our diets are adequate and provide these nutrients in good balance.

Less Salt in Hypertension

Food labels, which show nutrients in the order of their health implications, list sodium right after fat, indicating we need to pay attention to how much sodium our diets provide. Salt or sodium chloride, one of the major sources of this nutrient, contains roughly half sodium and half chloride. The steady increase of salt in our diets during this century to excessive levels and its relationship with hypertension, a risk factor for heart disease, has led to a reevaluation of sodium nutrition.

Sodium is an essential nutrient, and our diet must provide some on a daily basis. For most individuals the daily sodium

154

intake can vary over a wide range without adverse reaction. However, when the salt intake becomes excessive, profound effects on water retention occur. The increased body burden of salt results in fluid retention. People feel bloated and the increased fluid in the circulation raises blood pressure. Conversely, low salt diets result in fluid loss from the body and a simultaneous moderate drop in blood pressure. This is the reason for reducing salt intake in hypertension. Low salt diets have sometimes been used for weight reduction, and dieters have experienced a spectacular drop in body weight upon switching from a high salt to a low salt diet. However, the weight loss under such conditions is only fluid (not fat), which returns with increased salt intake.

Table salt contains:

40 percent sodium

60 percent chloride

While the changes to moderate salt diets have some effects on blood pressure, the cause of hypertension is not well known. In addition to excess dietary sodium, other factors play a role—such as genetic predisposition, the amount of stress in a person's life, and nutritional factors other than sodium. Decreasing excessive life stresses, eating a variety of wholesome foods that provide calcium (from dairy products), potassium (from vegetables, fruits, potatoes), and controlling the sodium intake are all helpful.

Our total diet should provide not more than 2,400 mg sodium per day. (This is approximately equivalent to one level teaspoon full of table salt per day.) To plan diets with sodium intakes less than 2,400 mg, we first need to use the salt shaker judiciously or not at all. Furthermore, food label reading becomes a must because so many foods contain sodium and salt is added to innumerable food items. In addition to salt (sodium chloride), many other additives contain sodium, such as sodium monoglutamate (MSG) used as flavor enhancer in soups and many other food products, sodium bicarbonate (baking powder) in bakery products, sodium benzoate, sodium nitrate, and sodium nitrite used as preservatives in cold cuts, hot dogs, and many other foods. Many medications, even toothpastes, and drinking water may contain sodium.

Sodium Contents of Salts

One level teaspoon of	Sodium (mg)
Table salt	2,300
Celery salt	1,500
Garlic salt	2,020
Onion salt	1,400–1,500

The daily value (DV) is a reference value used on food labels to help consumers identify the relative contribution of a nutrient in a serving of the food to the total diet.

For sodium as well as total fat, saturated fat, and cholesterol, a lower-percentage DV is better than a high value.

Sodium is distributed widely in foods, and there is sufficient sodium naturally present in foods like milks, cheese, meats and chicken, most breads, and a host of prepared foods without adding more as table salt. Label reading is extremely important to identify foods high in sodium. In almost all cases, a food with lower sodium content can be substituted. Use fresh or frozen vegetables, naturally low in salt, rather than high-salt canned vegetables. Some foods are so high in sodium that they are better omitted or replaced by another similar, low-salt item. Many canned soups, all kinds of pickles, cured meats, cold cuts, hams, salted chips, and some sauces are high in salt. If you cook your own meals, use spices and herbs instead of salt to good advantage.

Some have claimed that Americans are addicted to salt, and indeed it takes only a few days to get hooked on high-salt diets. Once used to highly salted foods, a person needs to make a conscious effort to change from excess to a moderate-salt diet. But when we have adjusted to less salt, we feel better, less bloated and may actually develop a dislike for highly salted foods. On low-salt diets, we can taste the natural flavor of foods. We enjoy a food because of its unique flavor rather than the added salt. Eating daily a selection of fresh fruits and vegetables as suggested by the food guide will automatically reduce our sodium intake because these foods are low in sodium (but high in potassium). So if we follow the recommendations for healthful eating, by taking care of our whole diet, we will reduce our salt intake as a matter of course.

Finally, always keep in mind that sodium is an essential nutrient and too severe dietary sodium restriction should be avoided. At very low sodium intakes, our kidneys must work harder to conserve sodium, and in the wake of this conservation, a hormone is produced (angiotensin), which can drive blood pressure even higher. Under certain conditions sodium-restricted diets may have even detrimental effects. The hypertension of pregnancy toxemia, for example, calls for salt and fluid given under medical supervision. Another case is prolonged physical exercise, especially in hot weather. Liberal salt and fluid intake are required to counteract the salt and water loss during excessive sweating, which can result in heat stroke.

Raise Calcium in Osteoporosis

Calcium together with phosphorus makes up bone and teeth. They are also necessary for many other functions in the body. When dietary intake of calcium is low, calcium is released from bone to cover these needs. To prevent excessive calcium loss from bone and to keep bone healthy, a sufficient daily intake of calcium is necessary. Dairy products are the best dietary sources of calcium and two to three cups of milk (use the low-fat kind) will cover the daily adult requirement of calcium. An exception is butter or cream, which are devoid of calcium. For the efficient absorption of calcium from the gut, vitamin D is also required. In the United States, milk is fortified with vitamin D to get this benefit.

Table 16

Some High Calcium Foods

Type of Food	Amount	Calcium (mg)
Milk, skim	1 cup	296
Milk, whole	1 cup	288
Yogurt	1 cup	294
Kidney beans, cooked	1 cup	204
Ice cream	1 cup	194
Salmon	3 oz	162
American cheese	1 slice	132
Spinach	1/2 cup	116
Rhubarb	1/2 cup	105
Cottage cheese	4 oz	102

(Note: There is no calcium in cream.)

From Food Composition Tables from Bowes and Church Composite

Osteoporosis is the gradual loss of bone during aging. The National Institute of Health estimates that 15 million people in the United States suffer from osteoporosis and that one out of four women with osteoporosis suffers bone fractures. Everybody loses some bone mass during aging. Women are more susceptible to osteoporosis for the simple reason that they usually have a smaller skeleton than men. Men also get osteoporosis, but it takes longer for their skeleton to get depleted of calcium. Another reason is that women are protected from bone loss by estrogen. After menopause their bone loss may be greatly accelerated and eventually the bone gets so thin that fractures and severe bone disease occur.

Nine Characteristics of People Most Likely to Get Osteoporosis

They are female   don't exercise
are Caucasian or Asian   often diet
are postmenopausal   drink too much alcohol
have small bones   smoke too much
don't drink milk

What can be done to lessen the severity of bone loss with aging? If you start with a big skeleton formed during adolescence, you are ahead in this game. Adequate calcium intakes during growth help to develop bone mass. This is the first prerequisite. During adulthood keeping active is also very helpful. Exercise keeps the calcium in bone and will retard bone loss. And of course you need to get your daily calcium. The National Osteoporosis Foundation recommends 1,500-mg elemental calcium for post-menopausal women who are not on hormone replacement. A total of 1,500 mg (1.5 gram) would be the amount of calcium in about five cups of milk. Such high calcium intakes are best obtained partly by diet (two servings of 1 percent milk provide 600-mg calcium) and partly from a calcium supplement.

What to Do to Lessen Osteoporosis

Eat a nutritionally adequate diet
Practice moderation: prevent too much dietary protein, alcohol, and fiber
Exercise to strengthen your bones: walk, jog, or bike regularly
Get vitamin D from some sunshine exposure, and/or from vitamin supplements
Consider taking a calcium supplement
Postmenopausal women may consider estrogen replacement
Stop smoking

Hypertension, a risk factor for heart disease, is another disorder that is influenced by dietary calcium. Several types of studies have associated hypertension to suboptimal calcium intake. Data obtained by the National Health and Nutrition Examination Survey (HANES I) have shown that individuals with hypertension had 8 to 20 percent lower dietary calcium intakes than individuals with "normal" blood pressure. In another study, blood pressure decreased after providing 1,000-mg dietary calcium per day to individuals with hypertension.

Approximately three-fourths of the daily calcium in American diets is obtained from dairy foods, such as milk, yogurt, cottage cheese and other cheeses. Green leafy vegetables such as collards, kale, bok choy, and turnip greens are good calcium sources from vegetables (but cook them in little water to retain the calcium). A serving of sardines with bones provides as much calcium as a cup of milk. Many other foods, and sometimes drinking water, if it is hard water, contain some calcium. Many mixed dishes to which either milk or cheese has been added contribute to our calcium intake. For efficient calcium absorption from the diet, vitamin D obtained from diet and/or sun exposure of our skin is necessary. Factors that depress calcium absorption from diet are excessive intakes of fiber and phosphorus. Phosphorus is added to many soft drinks, and the excessive use of such drinks can overload our diet. If we eat balanced diets, the effects of fiber and phosphorus in relation to calcium are minimal.

35–40% Americans get too much phosphorus in their diet. Too much phosphorus increases loss of calcium from bone. Most of the extra phosphorus comes from soft drinks and some other food.
—D. Anderson et al., "Dietary Phosphorus: The Benefits and the Problems," *Nutrition Today* 29 (1994): 29–34.

Calcium supplements are helpful, if calcium intakes greater than the RDA of 800 mg are recommended as for the prevention of osteoporosis or if dairy products are not tolerated. Many calcium preparations are on the market, which vary in their calcium content, their absorption efficiency from the gut, and their cost. Calcium from oyster shells, dolomite, and bone meal are not recommended because of possible contamination with metals such as lead or cadmium.

Table 17

Percent Calcium in Calcium Supplements

Type	% Calcium	Remarks
Calcium carbonate	40	
Tricalcium phosphate	38	contains phosphorus
Dicalcium phosphate	31	contains phosphorus
Bone meal	31	may contain contaminants
Calcium orange juice (*Citrus Hill Plus*)	30	part of a food
Oyster shell	28	may contain contaminants
Dolomite	22	may contain contaminants
Calcium citrate	21	
Calcium levulinate	13	
Calcium lactate	13	
Calcium gluconate	9	

—Based on data published by D.L. Levenson and R.S. Backman. "A Review of Calcium Preparations," *Nutrition Review* 52 (7) (1994): 221–232.

Children and adults with milk intolerance may not drink milk, and their calcium intake may be deficient. Milk intolerance is suspected if milk consumption regularly results in stomach-ache, cramps, and diarrhea. It can be due either to a milk protein allergy or to the inability to break down the milk sugar. Allergy to milk often occurs early in life and flares up when infants are weaned from mother's to cow's milk. Sometimes goat or soy milk can be substituted without ill effects. Milk intolerance due to the inability to digest the milk sugar "lactose" is comparatively common in black children and in people of Asian and Mediterranean origin. In lactose intolerance, the milk sugar is not digested;

instead it is fermented by gut bacteria and the gas and acids thus produced result in gastrointenstinal upsets and painful cramps. These ill effects are prevented by choosing dairy products with very low lactose content, such as yogurt and some cheeses. Addition of the enzyme *lactose* to milk predigests the milk sugar and makes milk safe for children with lactose intolerance.

Iron and the Anemia Connection

Iron is needed for the hemoglobin of red blood cells, which carries oxygen from the lungs to brain, muscles and other body cells. Too little iron in the diet, or accelerated iron loss as during chronic bleeding over time, results in iron deficiency anemia with decreased oxygen available to our tissues. When our body cells are oxygen-starved, the energy in our dietary fat and carbohydrate is not used efficiently. Therefore, the iron-deficient, anemic person is constantly tired, irritable, and gets exhausted upon the slightest exertion. Iron supplements will cure this type of anemia in a matter of weeks. However, it is better to prevent the anemia in the first place.

Iron deficiency anemia is the most common form of anemia. A simple blood test will tell the cause of tired blood and what needs to be done about it.

Good dietary iron sources are red meats, liver, egg, dried fruits, and green leafy vegetables. The major problem with dietary iron is its low bioavailability. The absorption from the gut is quite low and on averge only 5 to 10 percent of the dietary iron is absorbed and utilized. Iron absorption can be increased in several ways:

1. We can select a food from which iron absorption is more efficient. The iron in red meat (as heme iron) is absorbed with an improved efficiency. Since balanced

diets include some meats, we will get part of our iron need from this source.

2. Another way to increase the intestinal absorption of dietary iron is to mix foods that increase the efficiency of iron absorption. Vitamin C from citrus fruit and other sources increases the intestinal absorption of vegetable and cereal iron. If you eat an orange or have a glass of orange juice with your iron-fortified cereal in the morning, you will absorb more of the iron from the cereal. Vitamin C has no effect on the absorption of meat iron.

3. Several foods interfere with iron absorption. Milk depresses iron absorption from foods and from iron pills. Some nutritionists have suggested eating dairy foods and iron-rich foods at different meals. However, we do not understand the interactions of foods during digestion sufficiently to make such recommendations.

4. We can increase the amount of iron ingested as from iron supplements, which are somewhat better absorbed than the majority of food iron. Given in doses equivalent to the RDA, such supplements can be helpful for individuals at risk for iron-deficiency anemia.

However, we need to keep in mind that anemia (tired blood) can be due to causes other than iron deficiency. For example, a deficiency of vitamin B_{12}, or of folate, results also in anemia. To distinguish between the different kinds of anemias, a simple blood test is used so that the proper treatment is selected. Iron deficiency anemia is cured and prevented only by iron, while the anemia due to folate and/or vitamin B_{12} deficiency requires folate and vitamin B_{12} for treatment. Once iron deficiency is determined and iron supplements are taken, the red blood cells return to normal and the anemia clears up within weeks. However, further iron is needed to build up iron stores in the liver, which are necessary for proper immune function. Low iron states that may occur even before iron-deficiency anemia is diagnosed result in lowered ability to fight infections. Population groups such as women, preschool children, growing adolescents, and individuals with chronic blood loss are especially prone to low iron status.

Groups of People Most Likely to Have Tired Blood

Children between three and five years of age
Teenage girls and boys
Women of child-bearing age
Individuals with chronic low-level blood loss

Fluoride and Better Teeth

When infinitesimally small amounts of fluoride are incorporated into our tooth enamel during tooth formation, our teeth are more resistant to tooth decay throughout life. Once our teeth are formed without incorporated fluoride, this protection is lost even though fluoride treatments and fluoridated toothpastes have some lesser benefits.

Our diets contain variable amounts of fluoride. However, dictary fluoride is tightly bound to food and appears not available for tooth formation. Fluoride dissolved in drinking water on the other hand in concentrations of 0.8 to 1 microgram per ml has been shown to protect from tooth decay. Fluoride is naturally present in many U.S. water supplies, and children growing up in these areas are remarkably free of tooth decay. Because of the well-proven benefit of fluoride, communities that have no or too little fluoride in drinking water may add fluoride to drinking water. Fluoridation of public drinking water has had a spectacular success in the prevention of caries and tooth decay.

Iodine and Goiter

Throughout human history iodine deficiency has been a problem, especially in mountainous areas where plants and water are low in iodine. In the Andes of South America and the Alps of Switzerland, for example, iodine deficiency was so severe that not only adults had the unsightly enlargements of the thyroid gland in the neck, but children became physically and mentally stunted due to iodine deficiency. That the lack of a single nutrient can alter so radically a person's growth and development is truly remarkable and shows the importance of providing all essential nutrients.

In the absence of iodine, the thyroid cannot make its hormone, causing hypothyroidism. All body processes slow down, less energy is used, and more fat is deposited in adipose tissue. This is why hypothyroid people become easily obese. Hypothyroidism also affects the brain. Mentation becomes sluggish and people think and move slowly.

Only a fraction of a milligram (0.150 mg) of iodine is needed daily; yet if this small amount is absent from the diet, deficiency of iodine eventually occurs. Seafood is the best source of dietary iodine and vegetables grown near the oceans are also good sources because the rains carry iodine-containing water to nearby agricultural lands. The small amount of iodine in iodized salt has prevented goiter in generations of the Midwestern U.S. population and in many peoples around the globe.

Seafood is the best source of dietary iodine. If for any reason you do not eat any seafood, use iodine-fortified salt—sparingly.

One problem today is that we sometimes get more iodine than we really need. Sources of contamination are jodophors used as industrial cleaning compounds, iodine-containing cough medicine, seaweed vegetables, and several others. Too much iodine interferes with the uptake of iodine into the thyroid gland and consequently decreases the synthesis of thyroid hormone. The end result is also a goiter. This is one of the unusual situations when too little or too much of a nutrient produces the same devastating end effects.

Zinc—Last but Not Least

Zinc is often regarded as the last in the long list of nutrients. Although no specific "Disease of Civilization" has been identified due to imbalance of this nutrient, it is as critical for well-being as any other essential nutrient. Adequate dietary zinc intake is required for speedy wound healing, for example. Low zinc states have contributed to growth stunting in children on poor diets, to sickness in alcoholics, to cardiovascular disease and even cancer, among others. Good dietary sources of zinc are meat, milk, and whole grains, while fruits and vegetables contribute lesser amounts. Mixed, wholesome diets are most likely to provide adequate levels of zinc.

Overall Mineral Adequacy

In the above sections, we have mentioned only several of the twenty or so essential mineral elements that our diet must provide. Since these nutrients come from different food groups and different foods within each group, eating a variety of foods from each group becomes mandatory. Variety in your food selection is necessary and will most likely provide for your need of minerals and reduce the chance of either deficiency or toxicity. Even though for some of these nutrients little data exist to relate them to specific chronic disease states, all mineral nutrients are vital for good health. Just consider magnesium, required for practically all energy transformations in the human body. If we want to utilize the energy in carbohydrates and fats, magnesium is an obligatory nutrient that must be present. Or consider potassium, required by each of our body cells, with specific functions in nerve transmission and vital for the pacemaker of our heart. We obtain magnesium from whole grains, legumes, and green leafy vegetables (as part of the green chlorophyll) and potassium from fruits and vegetables. Highly refined foods are usually poor sources of both these nutrients. Variety in your diet again is the key, and good magnesium and potassium nutrition is a "byproduct" of choosing a diet of whole grains and legumes, green leafy vegetables, and fresh fruits.

One yet unresolved question regarding some trace mineral elements is their varying amounts in foods, reflecting the environmental conditions under which foods are grown. An example is the antioxidant nutrient selenium, which we obtain predominantly from wheat. Luckily for us, most wheat in the United States is produced on the high-selenium Midwestern soils and therefore is a good source of this nutrient. A similar situation occurs for iodine, which is higher in foods produced near the oceans as compared to inland areas. Eating a variety of foods, grown under different conditions, can even out such differences due to environmental factors and, is the best policy for adequate and safe intakes of these nutrients.

Step Twelve: Your Dietary Mineral Nutrients

Variety in our food selection as suggested all along is necessary for our diet to obtain all mineral elements. The mineral nutrients we should limit are sodium from table salt and processed foods and phosphorus, which is added to many soft drinks among other sources. Excess intakes of trace minerals from supplements can be dangerous and must be prevented. Higher than usual intakes, medically indicated for specific reasons, should be given under a physician's care.

The following will guide you through the maze of mineral nutrition. Check how you are doing:

1. First be sure you receive per day **at least** the following:
   - Six grain servings, at least half of the whole-grain type
   - Three vegetable servings low in salt
   - Two fruit servings with low sugar content
   - Two of the milk/dairy servings—low-fat types
   - Five servings of the meat group

167

      If yes —— good

      If no —— go back to earlier chapters to improve your overall nutrition

2. Do you make heavy use of the salt shaker?

      If no —— good

      If yes —— cut down

3. Do you read labels for sodium content of foods?

      If yes —— good

      If no —— start now, select foods with low % DV for sodium

4. Do you substitute low-sodium food for high-sodium foods?

      If yes —— good

      If no —— substitute foods with lower % DV

5. Do you suffer from hypertension? Get medical advice regarding your sodium intake.

6. If you are at risk for osteoporosis, you might want to consider calcium supplements, *not to replace,* but in addition to your two servings of dairy foods per day.

7. If you are at risk for osteoporosis, limit soft drinks with high phosphorus content. Excess phosphorus depletes your bone calcium.

8. American mixed diets provide approximately six milligrams of iron per 1,000 Cals per day. This iron may not be sufficient for individuals at risk for iron-deficiency anemia. If you feel run down and are in that category, have it checked out by a physician. A one-a-day iron supplement may be helpful.

9. If you are on a weight-reduction diet and you consume a low-calorie diet, you must supplement your diet with a one-a-day-type vitamin/mineral supplement, even if you consume a nutrient-dense diet.

In conclusion just consider the following points in relation to your mineral nutrition:

- The meat group should be limited because of the saturated fat, but if we limit too much, we lose good sources of iron and zinc.
- Salt should be limited, but too severe restriction eliminates an important source of dietary iodine if you get most of your iodine from iodized salt.
- Your calcium intake is likely to be too low if your diet omits dairy foods.
- If you include too many processed foods, your diet may provide too much sodium.

From the few examples, it is clear that dietary balance is of paramount importance. Whenever we digress from eating balanced diets, we automatically affect a variety of nutrients. Any extreme diet is undesirable. Balance is the key. We are meant to eat and enjoy a variety of food. Balanced diets as suggested by the food guide are the best way to obtain all nutrients, including minerals, vitamins, protein, fiber, and calories from carbohydrates and fat in adequate and safe amounts for good health.

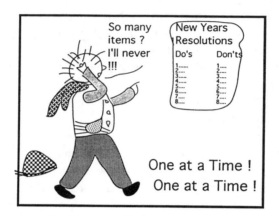

Chapter XIV
Some Ifs and Buts of Eating

I Eat What I Like

Food is not only a necessity, a provider of life-giving nutrients and energy but also a source of pleasure, relaxation, and gratification. Meal times for most people are a welcome interruption from the daily grind. Eating on the run, not taking time to sit down and enjoy one's food, may deprive a person of some of these benefits. Even if your time for meals is limited, your food selection can and should be nutritious, pleasing, and psychologically satisfying.

It helps if you have come to like healthful food. At present we know far too little of why one person will drool over steak while another may dislike it. Our food likes and dislikes are highly individual. Even siblings, raised in exactly the same environment may have vastly different taste preferences. One may like fatty and another only lean meats! Innumerable such examples could be cited. From studies with newborns, we know that some taste preferences are inborn. Placing several drops of a sugar solution on the tongue of newborns who had never tasted any food before made them smile, while a bitter solution made them grimace. However, most of our food preferences are acquired during childhood. Getting used to different kinds of foods is a learning process superimposed on our physiological taste and flavor preferences. A new food, unknown to a person, may be automatically disliked. Intense food dislikes can be induced by eating a food during an episode of nausea, for example. Subconsciously, the food is associated with feeling sick and this may induce a strong dislike for the food. Conversely, a food that you associate with feeling good will help you to like this food.

From a health point of view, many different diets can provide good nutrition. The person who by choice or upbringing has learned to like foods that provide optimum health has a great advantage over somebody who does not care. Man has an uncanny ability to like the familiar; the Australian Aborigine may feast on grasshoppers, the Italian on pasta, and modern youth on hamburger and french fries. There is nothing wrong with eating what one likes, but it is absolutely necessary to look at one's food habits to see whether or not they are health-giving. One of the best investments is the introduction of a healthful lifestyle, with variable, balanced, and moderate diets, which taste good and are liked. The trick is to like what's good for us.

Sinful Foods

Probably everybody likes one or several foods that should not be part of our diet on a regular basis. The food may be too high in calories, may contain too much fat, may be too salty, or may provide too many empty calories. Cutting it out completely may backfire and lead to strong cravings hard to resist.

Everybody can have an occasional sinful food. If strong cravings occur, the person must plan his/her diet with care. Satisfying diets with regular meals usually decrease excessive hunger cravings. If the craving is for a specific food, eat it at the end of a meal when your hunger is satisfied. Cravings may occur at specific times of the day when confronted with the grind of daily problems. To know what sets off a particular craving is helpful so that the source can be eliminted or strategies may be developed to minimize the food craving. The portion size of a sinful food also needs to be considered. To get used to smaller sized portions, substituting the food occasionally for another regular item in the diet, or expending more energy (if it is a high-calorie food), all are helpful ways.

Above all keep the total diet in mind. When the splurging food displaces too many regular food items, especially vegetables, fruits, and the like, one must make sure it does not get out of hand. Only buying a small amount of the sinful food or keeping it fairly inaccessible are strategies that sometimes work. Eating the particular food in company, rather than eating alone when it is easy to lose all sense of proportion, can be helpful. It is all right to pamper oneself, but remember you decide how to do it. If it gets out of hand, find out the underlying reasons. To solve problems by eating does not serve any purpose. The price one pays by using food to make oneself feel better can be enormous.

Addiction to Food

A good meal makes one feel good, and it is no secret that when things go wrong in one's life, food can give a certain gratification that makes trouble more bearable. Going without food for a while makes one feel empty, the stomach starts growling, and painful hunger pangs are felt. When this happens food is constantly on one's mind, and automatically or consciously people look for food. The reasons for the feeling of hunger and the effect of hunger on human behavior are very complex, and we have no good explanation of their workings. That the brain, at least in part, controls them is well documented. Of great interest is the discovery that food intake regulation and emotions are both influenced by the hypothalamus—a specific area in the brain. This may explain in part that emotions affect our food behaviors and vice versa. However, for compulsive food behaviors, such as the self-imposed abstinence from food in anorexia nervosa, or the compulsive overeating as in bulimia, we have at present no explanation of the causes of such aberrant behavior. While these disorders have serious nutritional consequences, their causes are believed primarily psychological. Rehabilitation must direct the therapy at the underlying causes and at the same time deal with the nutritional implications.

Eating Out

Not long ago practically everybody, except travellers, had their meals at home. Today this has radically changed and many people take more meals away from home than at their dining-room table. By eating out we have innumerable options; fast foods, specialty foods, ethnic foods, fully prepared meals to take to the workplace, are only a few that are offered to the public. With the ever greater selection of convenience foods, individuals traditionally involved in food preparation in the home are turning to other occupations.

In former times it was the job of women to make sure the farm produced enough food to prepare nourishing meals for the family. Today with the disintegration of the conventional family, urban life, and individualized lifestyles, more people need to make their own decisions about food. Consequently, knowledge of foods and how to select nutritious diets is necessary for practically every adult. Food eaten out needs to be chosen with the same care as home-style fare, and the total diet must be considered. If you eat lunch in a fast food place without any vegetables, you must choose vegetables at the following meal. One of the difficulties is that in many cases we do not know the ingredients—such as the type of fat, the amount of salt or sugar present in a food. For fat-controlled diets, it is usually safe to eat vegetables plain and meats without or with little gravy and to use the salt shaker only after tasting the food.

The food industry has been receptive to modern requests for low calorie, low fat, and low salt foods. These products are also used by restaurants and fast food places. But although such trends have become popular, many food items served in restaurants are still high in fat, salt, and empty calories. To select nutritious food, keep the food pyramid in mind. Ask what the ingredients are in a dish, ask for low-salt items, ask for vegetables, and ask for low-fat items. If you eat out once in a blue moon, you can splurge and even out excess or deficiency at your next meal. However, if you eat out regularly, you must start selecting foods that are enjoyable and good for your health (see figure 13).

Ethnic Foods

The United States is a melting pot in more than one way. The people who have emigrated from all parts of the globe brought with them their traditions and also their specific diets. Some kept their food habits, and we talk of Italian, Greek, Jewish, Japanese, Chinese, Indian, Mexican, soul food among many others while yet others have acculturated to eat conventional American diets.

174

Rate Your Plate when Eating Out

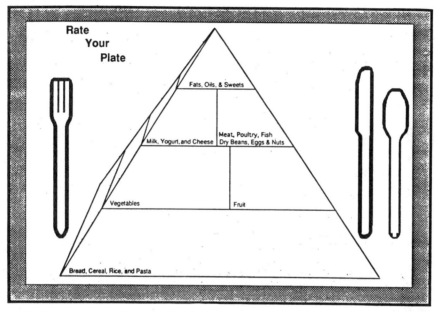

Taken from the 1993 Pyramid Packet, Penn State Nutrition Center, University Park, PA 16801.

Figure 13

Each of these groups has its own food specialties, food likes and dislikes.

All through human history, people's food habits were determined by traditions, religious beliefs, taboos, and by economic considerations of food availability. Thus food habits evolved, were handed down from generation to generation, and eventually have become entrenched in a culture. All major religions had traditions related to food, and the evolution of ethnic foods was observed globally. In the United States some ethnic and religious groups still follow their old food traditions while others have broken with them and have adopted new ways and ideas.

The search for new lifestyles in the United States has been influenced by the idea of individuality and self-determination. Everybody needs to work out his/her own lifestyle in a rapidly changing world. Some do it by imitation, some by trial and error, some reason it out, and others are just lucky to fall into a lifestyle that is healthful and satisfying. Most of us, though, to develop a lifestyle conducive to health and well-being, must painstakingly learn what is best. While the tradition-bound person learned from early childhood what was expected and allowed, modern people must learn for themselves and this learning process is often slow and painful.

If you follow an ethnic food tradition, such as Italian or Chinese, for example, you need to review your own practices to see whether they are in line with healthful eating. The changes you need to make may be small; perhaps you'll need to change your cooking fat, or include more vegetables, or simply alter the food portions you usually serve. Compare what you do with the recommendations of the food guide. If need be, cook creatively and change a food recipe to a more healthful dish. Ethnic foods have developed over time as an adaptation to specific conditions, and you should feel free to continue this adaptation if need be so that the food you eat will give you the maximum health benefit.

Beware of Extreme Diet

Any extreme diet is harmful if followed over extended time. Well-planned vegetarian diets are well tolerated by adults, but children need some foods of animal origin, like milk and meat, or they become growth stunted. Fruitarians, piscaterians, meat and potato eaters, dieters, fasters, milk omitters, fletcherizers, macrobiotics, snackers on empty calories, fast food eaters, etc., who shun foods from one or several food groups put themselves at risk. The longer imbalanced diets are consumed, the more acute these imbalances become. Inadequate nutrition proceeds from suboptimal nutrient levels in the body to changes in subtle and then pronounced function and eventually to frank disease. Examples are:

Diets omitting the milk/dairy group partially or completely during the adolescent growth spurt result in a smaller skeleton and likelihood of osteoporosis in later life. Low-calcium intakes also lead to greater lead absorption from environmental sources and the risk of lead toxicity in children.

Diets limiting vegetable and fruit intake will be low in several vitamins and antioxidants as well as fiber. This increases the risk for several cancers, may predispose to diverticular disease and free radical damage associated with a series of disorders.

Diets that provide excessive amounts of refined foods are too high in empty calories. They may predispose a person to obesity and at the same time to vitamin and mineral deficiencies. Examples of such imbalances abound. We need to remember that our body works best when we eat mixed diets, which provide nutrients in variety, balance, and moderation. We are essentially omnivores, with strong tendencies to require vegetables and fruits within the framework of our total diet.

The Game of Dieting

What has been written and advertised about dieting would fill volumes of books. Money spent on slimming diets and slenderizing potions could feed an army with wholesome food. It is not immediately obvious why many of these diet attempts fail. As the causes of obesity are many, so are also the reasons for failure. One thing is clear: the success rate for slimming is disappointing and failure is unfortunately the order of the day. There is no easy answer. But in most cases two major points are not taken into account. The first is the underlying cause of obesity is not dealt with and the second is the resentment to change one's lifestyle—increasing activity and putting diet on the right course. Without understanding the energy that drives us to do what we do, food will be always at the beck and call of these hidden drives. Sugar may compensate for lack of love, overeating may help to forget hurtful disappointments, or binging on a high calorie food may dispel boredom. To confront squarely and honestly the underlying cause(s) of obesity requires courage and honesty, but it is the first necessary step for change. Once this step is taken, diet and lifestyle can be tackled from the right perspective. To improve your diet is less threatening because your attitude has changed and food habits are not driven by this unknown force.

To get your weight-loss diet on the right track, you must first review your present diet as proposed in earlier chapters. This will give you a baseline from which to start. From now on plan your diet carefully. Use the food guide and eat a diet that provides the recommended servings (select the lowest energy level without added fat that will give you a diet of approximately 1,200 to 1,300 Cal per day). This is a low-calorie diet, which provides a good balance of nutrients. Distribute the servings throughout the day to prevent excessive hunger feelings. Start out with breakfast. To prevent excessive hunger periods, you must not skip meals. It is important to get the required nutrients and only limit calories. Regular meals prevent excessive food cravings, which are apt to wreck a slimming program.

In addition, start exercising. If you have never exercised, walking for thirty minutes twice every day is a good start. If you can run, jog for a mile and increase the distance slowly at successive days. Both increased exercise and calorie restriction are necessary for a good weight reduction program. Exercise will start burning the fat in your adipose tissue, and the reduced dietary calories enhance this process. If you have a long way to go in your weight reduction program, you may get tired. Give yourself a holiday by keeping the status quo for a week or so—still going for walks but liberalizing your diet a bit, keeping your body weight at a constant level. Such a period will familiarize you with the diet you require for maintenance of a healthy body weight. When you are ready, start another period of strict eating and exercise to shed another few pounds.

The overall objective of weight reduction program is not primarily to shed poundage but to be healthier. Some individuals are naturally big, and unrealistic expectations are not called for. A program that leaves you tired, depressed, and discouraged does little for you. We must learn to enjoy healthful food and take pride putting good meals together that can sustain our health throughout life. No crash diet giving a quick fix is the answer. Insight about our human nature and about what makes us tick combined with a fair amount of mental work, careful planning, and knowledge about foods are needed for a chance to accomplish this.

Starting a Slimming Diet

For exercise, start walking. Plan to walk half an hour in the morning and half an hour in the afternoon. Keep that up on a steady schedule. Make sure you wear a good pair of walking shoes and comfortable clothes. Write down the time you walk every day and how long.

In addition plan a low-calorie diet. Use the food guide. Keep fat low but include some oil for the polys.

Table 18

Example of a Low-Calorie Diet Plan (Servings)

Grains:	2 at breakfast, lunch, and supper
Vegetables:	1 for lunch, 2 for supper
Fruit	1 for breakfast, 1 for lunch, 1 for snack
Dairy:	1 for breakfast, 1/2 for lunch, 1/2 for snack
Meat:	1 for breakfast, 2 for lunch, 2 for supper
Sugar/fat	only a little jam, maybe a pat of margarine or mayo, 1 teaspoon of oil
Alcohol:	none

Day One

Breakfast

brewed coffeé	2 cups
milk 1% fat	0.25 cup
scrambled egg/milk/marga.	1
oatmeal bread	2 slices
margarine (60% soft spread)	1 tbs
orange juice, reconst.	6 oz

Snack

yogurt low fat/fruit	1 cup

Lunch

noodles/enriched/salt	1 cup
chicken curried	2 oz
romaine lettuce, chopped	0.5 cup
spinach, chopped, raw	0.5 cup
low-cal Italian dressing	1 tb
peaches in light syrup	0.5 cup

Supper

chicken rice soup	1 cup
tuna salad	2.5 oz
mixed grain bread	2 slices
grapes Thompson	2 oz
tea herb	2 cups

Snack

milk or yogurt 1% fat	1 cup

Day Two

Breakfast

brewed coffee	2 cups
milk 1% fat	0.25 cup
oatmeal cooked (water/salt)	0.5 cup
milk 1% fat	0.5 cup
orange, Florida	1
whole-wheat bread	1 slice
jelly	1 packet

Lunch

minestrone soup	1 cup
pizza cheese, 1/8th of a 15" diameter	1 slice
butterhead lettuce, chopped	0.5 cup
Italian dressing, low cal	1 tsp

Supper

Sockeye salmon, baked	3 oz
yellow corn	0.5 cup
green beans	1 cup
white spring onions	0.25 cup
apple sauce	0.5 cup
vanilla ice milk, hard	0.25 cup

Snack

milk 1% fat	1 cup
banana	1

The two diets provide 1,323 and 1,326 Cal per day. Slight further calorie decreases by cutting the fat to the core (approximately 100 Cal per day less) would be possible without compromising nutrients. You could, for example, substitute skim milk and fat-free yogurt for the one percent milk and substitute very lean meats. It is important, though, to eat the recommended servings from the food groups and to distribute the foods in a regular meal plan throughout the day to prevent excessive hunger episodes. Prevent fasting and stick to your plan. Keep your snack for the time when you most need it.

Keep an eye on your body weight and weigh yourself, perhaps twice per month or weekly. Follow your exercise program, and plan your own low calorie diets using the servings from the food guide. The good point about following the food guide is that you have learned to eat diets that are good for life. Eventually, if you have obtained the desired weight, you can include more servings, starting first with servings from the vegetable and fruit group followed by more servings from the grain group.

Contemplating Change

Changes that affect our diet and lifestyle must be made gradually. Do not rush into a situation that makes things worse for you. Radical changes usually are difficult to sustain, as a pilot study to decrease the risk factors for heart disease has shown. Individuals in this study had to change their diets, stop smoking, and have their blood pressure treated all at the same time. The design of the study was impeccable, and much help was given the participants to assure a successful outcome. Unfortunately many individuals became depressed and the intervention had to be interrupted and modified. Too many changes, too fast, made the people in the study anxious and depressed.

We need to learn from a study like that to make changes step-wise lest we go too fast. People are different and what helps one may not work for another. Above all, a person must be ready to take responsibility for his/her own life. Unrealistic expectations lead to failure. Knowledge of oneself and what is good for one's body is the key. To apply the knowledge takes courage and perseverance. But in the end it is worth it.

APPENDICES

Appendix A
Further Reading

American Heart Association Kid's Cookbook. Ed. Mary Winston. New York: Times Books, 1993.

Bailey, Janet. *Keeping Food Fresh.* New York: Harper & Row, 1993.

Bowes and Church's Food Values of Portions Commonly Used. Revised by Jean A. T. Pennington. Philadelphia: J. B. Lippincott, 1994.

Callahan, Maureen. *Skimming the Fat: A Practical Food Guide.* The American Dietetic Association Item No 0810 (800/745-0775, Ext 5000).

Clark, Nancy. *Nancy Clark's Sport Nutrition Guidebook.* Leisure Press, 1990.

Consumer Report on Health. P.O. Box 53029, Boulder, CO 80322–3029.

Fat and Cholesterol Counter. American Heart Association. New York: Time Books/Random House, 1991.

FDA Consumer. Superintendent of Documents, Government Printing Office, Washington, DC 20402.

Health Counts: A Fat and Calorie Guide. Wiley: Kaiser Permanente, 1991.

Hess, Mary Abbott and Ann Elise Hunt. *Pocket Supermarket Guide.* The American Dietetic Association, 1989, Item No 0860. (800/745-0775, Ext 5000).

Lambert-Lagace, Louise. *Feeding Your Baby: From Conception to Age Two.* Surrey Books, 1991.

Nutrition Action Healthletter. Center of Science in the Public Interest, 1875 Connecticut Ave NW, Suite 300, Washington, DC 20009–5278.

Nutrition Today. Published bimonthly by Williams and Wilkins, 428 E. Preston Street, Baltimore, MD 21202.

Robertson, Laurel, Carol Flinders, Brian Ruppenthal. *Laurel's Kitchen Recipes.* Ten Speed Press, 1993.

Swinney, Bridget. *Eating Expectantly: The Essential Guide and Cookbook for Pregnancy.* Fall River: Fall River Press, 1993.

Tribole, Evelyn. *Eating on the Run.* Leisure Press, 1992.

Tufts University Diet & Nutrition Letter. 53 Park Place, New York, NY 10007.

University of California, Berkeley Wellness Newsletter. Health Letter Association, P.O. Box 420148, Palm Coast, FL 32142.

Appendix B
How to Estimate Your Daily Energy Needs

For the Healthy Adult Male

		Example
Needed:	Your Age:	30
	Your Body Weight in lbs:	155 lbs
	Your Height in inches:	72 inches

Multiply 6.2 times your weight in pounds	=	961
Multiply 12.5 times your height in inches	=	900
Add 66	=	66

TOTAL	=	1,927
Subtract 6.8 times your age in years	=	204
Your basal energy need in calories (BEE)	=	1,723 Cal

Select your lifestyle:

Sedentary (your BEE times 1.3)	=	2,240 Cal
Moderately active (your BEE times 1.5)	=	2,585 Cal
Extremely active (your BEE times 1.8)	=	3,100 Cal

The final figure is your approximate daily energy requirement.

Note: This is a very rough estimate. It does not apply if you are either severely underweight or obese. If underweight or obese, use your "desirable" body weight for the calculation.

For the Healthy Adult Female

		Example
Needed:	Your Age:	30
	Your Body Weight in lbs:	133 lbs
	Your Height in inches:	64 inches

Multiply 4.3 times your weight in pounds	=	572
Multiply 4.25 times your height in inches	=	272
Add 655	=	655

TOTAL	=	1,499
Subtract 4.7 times your age in years	=	141

Your basal energy need in calories (BEE)	=	1,358 Cal

Select your lifestyle:

Sedentary (your BEE times 1.3)	=	1,766 Cal
Moderately active (your BEE times 1.5)	=	2,038 Cal
Extremely active (your BEE times 1.8)	=	2,446 Cal

The final figure is your approximate daily energy requirement.

Note: This is a very rough estimate. It does not apply if you are either severely underweight or obese. If underweight or obese, use your "desirable" body weight for the calculation.

Appendix C

A Quick Way to Calculate Your Body Mass Index (BMI) for Men and Women

		Example:		
Needed:	Your body weight in Kg	weight 132 lbs		
	Your height in meters	height 64 inches		

Take your weight in pounds and divide it by 2.2. This will be your weight in kilograms	132/2.2	=	60 kg
Take your height in inches and multiply by 0.025. This will be your height in meters.	64 x 0.025	=	1.6 m
Square your height (in meters).	1.6 x 1.6	=	2.56
Your BMI = weight in kg/height in meter^2	60/2.56	=	23.4

A BMI greater than 27 is indicative of obesity.

A BMI between 24 and 27 is considered overweight for females.

A BMI between 24 and 25 is considered overweight for males.

Appendix D

Height and Weight Growth Charts for Children 2 to 18 Years of Age*

*Used with permission of Ross Products Division, Abbott Laboratories, Columbus, OH 4316. From *NCHS Growth Chts.,* © 1982 Ross Products Division, Abbot Laboratories.

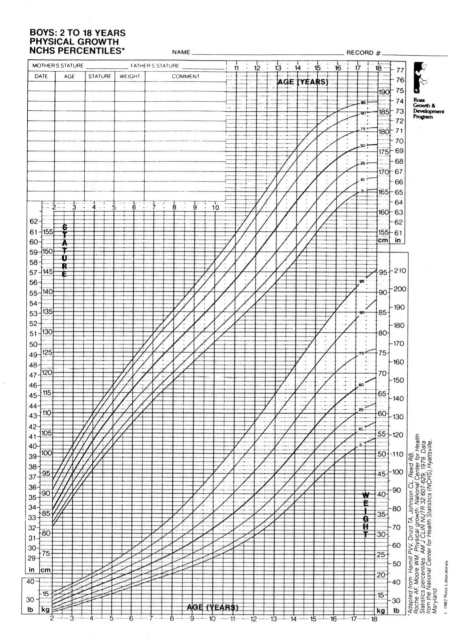

Figure 14

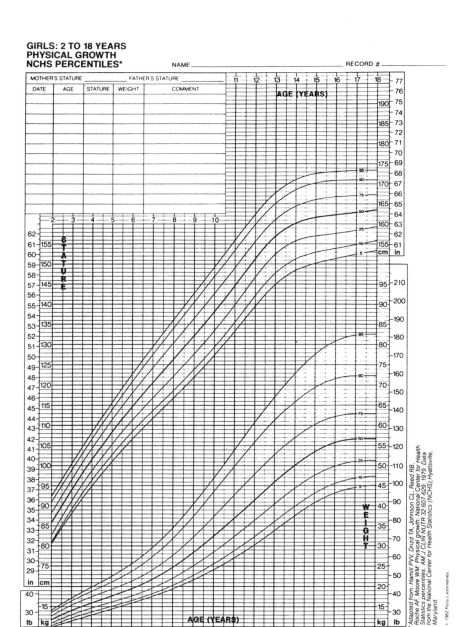

Figure 15

Appendix E
The Recommended Dietary Allowances

The recommended dietary allowances or RDAs are the nutrient amounts for maintenance of good nutrition of practically all healthy people in the United States. They are updated from time to time as new scientific data are obtained.

The daily value for vitamins and minerals on food labels (which is the same reference value as the old U.S. RDAs) is based on their respective RDAs.

The daily value for fat, saturated fat, total carbohydrate, dietary fiber, and protein varies with the calorie intake. The daily value for the energy nutrients are given on food labels for a 2,000-Cal diet. They must be adjusted upwards for higher calorie diets. For low-calorie diets, they need to be decreased.

FOOD AND NUTRITION BOARD, NATIONAL ACADEMY OF SCIENCES—NATIONAL RESEARCH COUNCIL

RECOMMENDED DIETARY ALLOWANCES,[a] Revised 1989

Designed for the maintenance of good nutrition of practically all healthy people in the United States

Category	Age (years) or Condition	Weight[b] (kg)	Weight[b] (lb)	Height[b] (cm)	Height[b] (in)	Protein (g)	Vita-min A (µg RE)[c]	Vita-min D (µg)[d]	Vita-min E (mg α-TE)[e]	Vita-min K (µg)	Vita-min C (mg)	Thia-min (mg)	Ribo-flavin (mg)	Niacin (mg NE)[f]	Vita-min B6 (mg)	Fo-late (µg)	Vitamin B12 (µg)	Cal-cium (mg)	Phos-phorus (mg)	Mag-nesium (mg)	Iron (mg)	Zinc (mg)	Iodine (µg)	Sele-nium (µg)
Infants	0.0–0.5	6	13	60	24	13	375	7.5	3	5	30	0.3	0.4	5	0.3	25	0.3	400	300	40	6	5	40	10
	0.5–1.0	9	20	71	28	14	375	10	4	10	35	0.4	0.5	6	0.6	35	0.5	600	500	60	10	5	50	15
Children	1–3	13	29	90	35	16	400	10	6	15	40	0.7	0.8	9	1.0	50	0.7	800	800	80	10	10	70	20
	4–6	20	44	112	44	24	500	10	7	20	45	0.9	1.1	12	1.1	75	1.0	800	800	120	10	10	90	20
	7–10	28	62	132	52	28	700	10	7	30	45	1.0	1.2	13	1.4	100	1.4	800	800	170	10	10	120	30
Males	11–14	45	99	157	62	45	1,000	10	10	45	50	1.3	1.5	17	1.7	150	2.0	1,200	1,200	270	12	15	150	40
	15–18	66	145	176	69	59	1,000	10	10	65	60	1.5	1.8	20	2.0	200	2.0	1,200	1,200	400	12	15	150	50
	19–24	72	160	177	70	58	1,000	10	10	70	60	1.5	1.7	19	2.0	200	2.0	1,200	1,200	350	10	15	150	70
	25–50	79	174	176	70	63	1,000	5	10	80	60	1.5	1.7	19	2.0	200	2.0	800	800	350	10	15	150	70
	51+	77	170	173	68	63	1,000	5	10	80	60	1.2	1.4	15	2.0	200	2.0	800	800	350	10	15	150	70
Females	11–14	46	101	157	62	46	800	10	8	45	50	1.1	1.3	15	1.4	150	2.0	1,200	1,200	280	15	12	150	45
	15–18	55	120	163	64	44	800	10	8	55	60	1.1	1.3	15	1.5	180	2.0	1,200	1,200	300	15	12	150	50
	19–24	58	128	164	65	46	800	10	8	60	60	1.1	1.3	15	1.6	180	2.0	1,200	1,200	280	15	12	150	55
	25–50	63	138	163	64	50	800	5	8	65	60	1.1	1.3	15	1.6	180	2.0	800	800	280	15	12	150	55
	51+	65	143	160	63	50	800	5	8	65	60	1.0	1.2	13	1.6	180	2.0	800	800	280	10	12	150	55
Pregnant						60	800	10	10	65	70	1.5	1.6	17	2.2	400	2.2	1,200	1,200	320	30	15	175	65
Lactating	1st 6 months					65	1,300	10	12	65	95	1.6	1.8	20	2.1	280	2.6	1,200	1,200	355	15	19	200	75
	2nd 6 months					62	1,200	10	11	65	90	1.6	1.7	20	2.1	260	2.6	1,200	1,200	340	15	16	200	75

[a] The allowances, expressed as average daily intakes over time, are intended to provide for individual variations among most normal persons as they live in the United States under usual environmental stresses. Diets should be based on a variety of common foods in order to provide other nutrients for which human requirements have been less well defined. See text for detailed discussion of allowances and of nutrients not tabulated.

[b] Weights and heights of Reference Adults are actual medians for the U.S. population of the designated age, as reported by NHANES II. The median weights and heights of those under 19 years of age were taken from Hamill et al. (1979) (see pages 16–17). The use of these figures does not imply that the height-to-weight ratios are ideal.

[c] Retinol equivalents. 1 retinol equivalent = 1 µg retinol or 6 µg β-carotene. See text for calculation of vitamin A activity of diets as retinol equivalents.

[d] As cholecalciferol. 10 µg cholecalciferol = 400 IU of vitamin D.

[e] α-Tocopherol equivalents. 1 mg d-α tocopherol = 1 α-TE. See text for variation in allowances and calculation of vitamin E activity of the diet as α-tocopherol equivalents.

[f] 1 NE (niacin equivalent) is equal to 1 mg of niacin or 60 mg of dietary tryptophan.

Permission to reproduce granted by National Academic Press, Washington, D.C. 20418.

Table 19

Summary Table. Estimated Safe and Adequate Daily Dietary Intakes of Selected Vitamins and Minerals [a] *

Vitamins

Category	Age (years)	Biotin (μg)	Pantothenic Acid (mg)
Infants	0–0.5	10	2
	0.5–1	15	3
Children and	1–3	20	3
adolescents	4–6	25	3–4
	7–10	30	4–5
	11+	30–100	4–7
Adults		30–100	4–7

Trace Elements[b]

Category	Age (years)	Copper (mg)	Manganese (mg)	Fluoride (mg)	Chromium (μg)	Molybdenum (μg)
Infants	0–0.5	0.4–0.6	0.3–0.6	0.1–0.5	10–40	15–30
	0.5–1	0.6–0.7	0.6–1.0	0.2–1.0	20–60	20–40
Children	1–3	0.7–1.0	1.0–1.5	1.0–2.5	20–80	25–50
	4–6	1.0–1.5	1.5–2.0	1.0–2.5	30–120	30–75
	7–10	1.0–2.0	2.0–3.0	1.5–2.5	50–200	50–150
	11+	1.5–2.5	2.0–5.0	1.5–2.5	50–200	75–250
Adults		1.5–3.0	2.0–5.0	1.5–4.0	50–200	75–250

[a]Because there is less information on which to base allowances, these figures are not given

[b]Since the toxic levels for many trace elements may be only several times usual intakes, the

*Reprinted with permission from RECOMMENDED DIETARY ALLOWANCES: 10TH EDITION. Copyright 1989 by the National Academy of Sciences. Courtesy of the National Academy Press, Washington, D.C.

Appendix F
Nutrient Content Claims*

Table 20

Nutrient	Free	Low	Reduced/Los	Comments
	Synonyms for "Free": "Zero," "No," "Without," "Trivial Source of," "Negligible Source of," "Dietarily insignificant Source of"	Synonyms for "Low": "Little," ("Few" for Calories), "Contains a Small Amount of," "Low Source of"	Synonyms for "Reduced"/"Less": "Lower" ("Fewer" for calories)	For "Free," "Very Low," or "Low," must indicate if food meets a definition without benefit of special processing; e.g., "broccoli, a fat-free food" or "celery, a low-calorie food"
Calories	Less than 5 calories per reference amount and per serving	40 calories or less per reference amount (and per 50 g if reference amount is small)	At lease 25% fewer calories per reference amount than an appropriate reference food. Uses term "Fewer" rather than "Less"	"Light" or "Lite:" if 50% or more of the calories are from fat, fat must be reduced by at lease 50% per reference amount. If less than 50% of calories are from fat, fat must be reduced at least 50% of calories or reduced at least 1/3 per reference amount
Total fat	Less than 0.5 g per reference amount and per serving*	3 g or less per reference amount (and per 50 g if reference amount is small)	At least 25% less fat per reference amount than an appropriate reference food	"____% Fat Free" must meet the requirements of "Low Fat"
Saturated fat	Less than 0.5 saturated fat and less than 0.5 *trans*-fatty acid per reference amount and per serving*	1 g or less per reference amount and 15% or less of calories from saturated fat	At least 25% less saturated fat per reference amount than an appropriate reference food	
Cholesterol	Less than 2 mg per reference amount and per serving*	20 mg or less per reference amount (and per 50 g if reference amount is small)	At least 25% less cholesterol per reference amount than an appropriate reference food	CHOLESTEROL CLAIMS ONLY ALLOWED WHEN FOOD CONTAINS 2 g OR LESS SATURATED FAT PER REFERENCE AMOUNT
Sodium	Less than 5 mg per reference amount and per serving*	140 mg or less per reference amount (and per 50 g if reference amount is small)†	At least 25% less sodium per reference amount than an appropriate reference food	"Light in Sodium": if food is reduced by at least 50% per reference amount. "Very Low Sodium:" 35 mg or less per reference amount (and per 50 g if reference amount is small). "Salt Free" must meet criterion for "Sodium Free"
Sugars	"Sugar Free": less than 0.5 g sugars per reference amount and per serving*	Not defined; no basis for a recommended intake	At least 25% less sugars per reference amount than an appropriate reference food	

*If an ingredient is present that is understood to contain this nutrient, it must be followed by an asterisk that refers to a footnote stating that it contains a trivial amount of the nutrient.

†"Small Reference Amount" = reference amount 30 g or less or 2 tablespoons or less.

*V. L. Wilkening, *Nutrition Today* 28 (57) (1993): 17, reprinted by permission.

Index